St. Louis Community College

Forest Park
Florissant Valley
Meramec

Instructional Resources
St. Louis, Missouri

Adolescence: An Ethological Perspective

Ritch C. Savin-Williams

Adolescence:
An Ethological Perspective

Springer-Verlag
New York Berlin Heidelberg London Paris Tokyo

Ritch C. Savin-Williams
Department of Human Development
  and Family Studies
Cornell University
Ithaca, NY 14853, U.S.A.

Library of Congress Cataloging-in-Publication Data
Savin-Williams, Ritch C.
  Adolescence: an ethological perspective.
  1. Adolescence. 2. Adolescent psychology.
3. Youth—Attitudes. I. Title.
HQ796.S287   1986   305.2'35   86-2033

Typeset by Ampersand Publisher Services Inc., Rutland, Vermont.
Printed and bound by R.R. Donnelley & Sons, Harrisonburg, Virginia.
Printed in the United States of America.

9 8 7 6 5 4 3 2 1

ISBN 0-387-96369-3 Springer-Verlag New York Berlin Heidelberg
ISBN 3-540-96369-3 Springer-Verlag Berlin Heidelberg New York

To *Francis Charles Williams* and
Joy Joan Savin Williams—they never
stopped loving

Preface

Books on adolescence have been written for a variety of purposes. Hall's (1904) two volume *Adolescence* encompasses most of them: to advocate a particular theoretical approach to adolescence, to stimulate use of a particular brand of scientific methodology when studying youth, to address issues of the basic nature and importance of adolescence, and to propose recommendations on how adolescents ought to be treated and educated. In Hall's words, "It [the two volumes] constitutes the first attempt to bring together the various aspects of its vast and complex theme" (xix), a full survey of "pedagogic matter and method." This is necessary because, "In no psychic soil, too, does seed, bad as well as good, strike such deep root, grow so rankly, or bear fruit so quickly or so surely" (xviii–xix).

Mead (1928) retorted with *Coming of Age in Samoa,* a refutation of Hall's conclusions: "Are the disturbances which vex our adolescents due to the nature of adolescence itself or to the civilization? Under different conditions does adolescence present a different picture" (p. 11). Thus, Mead wanted to correct a theoretical injustice and to promote the impact that culture has on the developing adolescent personality.

Hollingshead's (1949) *Elmtown's Youth* was produced to further support Mead's conclusions—"Is the social behavior of an adolescent a function of physiological changes in the maturing individual or of his experiences in society?" (p. 6). His answer was clearly the latter, specifically the family's economic and social status within Elmtown's social structure. Kiell (1964) countered both Mead and Hollingshead in *The Universal Experience of Adolescence:* "The present book attempts to demonstrate the universalities in adolescence as far back in history and in as many literate cultures as there are records" (p. 9). Inner turmoil and external behavioral disorder are characteristic of all adolescents and are "only moderately affected by cultural determinants" (p. 9).

Others joined the fray, writing supporting or contradicting books. The actors now strayed from the psychology versus sociology/anthropology disciplines to include historians, educators, ethologists, and social psychologists. For example, Kett (1977) wrote *Rites of Passage* to document the "polymorphism" of the social experience of youth, to trace the social forces and cultural moral values that have shaped youth, and to provide a historical perspective of the biases and distortions that have led to various societal responses to youth. The nature of adolescence and the causes of that nature have provided the major impetus for many of the most frequently cited books on adolescence. The goal is to present a more representative (Douvan & Adelson, 1966) or normal (Offer, 1969) sample of adolescents than that traditionally offered (e.g., Blos, 1962).

Books on adolescents may also serve to warn "society" of impending social doom unless the education of adolescents and their development are altered. Real adolescents are vanishing because they are being crushed by an insensitive adult world. Friedenberg (1959) wrote to describe adolescence as it is—a dumping ground for our cultural problems—and the way it should be: Adolescents need a clear and disciplined way of facing themselves and the world. In *The Adolescent Society* Coleman (1961) alerted parents and high schools that ignoring youth has resulted in a peer socialization process that severs adolescents from adult society and adult moral values. Schools should better implement the hopes and ideals of our society; if not, doom is inevitable.

Other books on adolescence were written to further a particular methodological approach. *The Jack Roller* (Shaw, 1930) illustrates how a delinquent boy's own subjective point of view of the events and sequences of social and cultural situations is essential to understand his life history, for both theoretical and therapeutic reasons. *Being Adolescent* (Csikszentmihalyi & Larson, 1984) promotes the Experience Sampling Method (paging device, beeper) as a technique of describing " ... what it is to be an adolescent from the inside, by letting teenagers tell us what they do, feel, and hope for as they go about their daily rounds ... " (p. xiv).

These theoretical, methodological, and moral exhortations are also addressed in the current volume. But, they do not constitute the major purpose. Rather, Thrasher (1927) stated the purpose best some 60 years ago in his preface to *The Gang:* "The Study is primarily an exploratory survey designed to reveal behavior-trends and to present a general picture of life in an area little understood by the average citizen. It is hoped that the book will encourage additional study in this field and indicate some interesting lines for further research" (p. xi). I would add, "little understood by the average researcher or theorist of adolescence."

My intent in writing this book is to share with you research that will provide an unfortunately rare perspective of adolescents and of adolescence. I make no claim that the participating adolescents are normal or representative of anything. There is no reliance on new methodological ploys; rather, psychology's most basic procedure, observations of behavior, is used. This method of yielding information emerges in a long-standing controversy; although most recognize that the naturalistic observation of behavior has merit, few engage in such activity. Finally, the research does not prove that adolescents are calm or conflicted or for what reason, whether physiological or cultural. But there is, to be honest, an orientation to emphasize the human typicality of adolescents and to interpret their behavior in an ethological, biological perspective. These points will be discussed further in Chapter 2.

The major personality and social issues addressed in this volume involve competitive and cooperative behavior among adolescents in naturalistic settings, with an emphasis on contextual, age, and sex variations. This interest began quite accidentally during my sophomore year in the psychology department at the University of Missouri. I was assigned to Dr. Robert Boice to assist with his research on dominance behavior among frogs. My task was to drop meal worms into pens of frogs, recording who ate when and who did what to whom. It was easy money in an air conditioned atmosphere inhabited by white rats, mice, marine toads, turtles, prairie dogs, and graduate students. But the job soon became an entry into scientific inquiry that was further developed in a biology of behavior class with Dr. Daniel G. Freedman in Human Development at the University of Chicago. Dr. Freedman's discussion of dominance hierarchy spanned many species but was limited, by virtue of the literature, to studies of children among humans. Yet, based on my experiences with adolescents at summer camp, the kinds of behaviors and structures discussed in the literature on frogs and children also appeared to characterize humans older than grade school age. My task was to document these impressions with a methodology based on observing behavior in naturalistic settings and with a theoretical perspective based on the tenets of ethology.

These views of methodology and development shaped the research and the analysis reported in this book. But I fear the data will do little to advance the field because of long-standing resistance of counter views. The studies are exploratory and they survey the range of adolescent competitive behaviors. They provide data that may be useful in a biosocial theoretical stance that incorporates an ethological perspective. Perhaps further research will be stimulated that will add more pieces to the picture of the natural adolescent's life.

I owe much gratitude to my fellow observers of adolescents, who also frequently served as co-authors of professional papers: Janet Bare Ashear, Joyce Canaan, Cathy Hannum, Birdy Paikoff, Debby Pool, Steve Small, Tom Spiegelhalter, Susan Spinola, Carol Walcer, and Shep Zeldin. The participating youth were always a joy to observe; in all cases they had the easiest task: to be themselves. A far more difficult task was to type the results of these observations. In this task Vicki Griffin was most dedicated, even discovering humor in the manuscript. When her fingers were bleeding profusely, Shawn Lovelace came to the rescue to spell her during times of healing. Colleagues assisted in a number of ways, from critical comments to statistical assistance. My thanks to Brad Brown, John Condry, Steve Cornelius, Mike Csikszentmihalyi, Gunhild Hagestad, Bob Johnston, Mort Lieberman, Martha McClintock, Don Omark, Rick Richards, Glenn Weisfeld and the many unnamed journal reviewers.

I suspect that much of the content of this book will seem commonplace, even obvious to you. If so, then it is confirmed that it borders on truth. For readers who have spent time with youth in contexts in which the youth choose to be, you will rediscover special memories, experiences, and knowledge. My attempt here is to recreate the obvious, for purposes of science and for those who educate youth. I want this book's major contribution to be the rekindling of knowledge and the rediscovery of an ancient behavioral science methodology. Perhaps you will welcome this book as an effort that you wished you had undertaken.

Contents

Preface vii

1 A Research Agenda 1
2 An Ethological Perspective on Dominance Behavior 17
3 Camp Wancaooah 37
4 Life in the Male Cabin Groups 51
5 Life in the Female Cabin Groups 81
6 Dominance Behaviors and Hierarchies in Male and Female
   Groups 105
7 Age as a Factor in Dominance and Social Behavior 131
8 Adolescent Altruism 157
9 Dominance and Altruism as Traits 173
10 Developing Perspective 189

Appendix A Early Adolescents 213
Appendix B Middle Adolescents 219

References 223
Author Index 237
Subject Index 243

1
A Research Agenda

As a graduate student at the University of Chicago in the early 1970s it was personally comforting but professionally disheartening to realize the ease with which one could claim that he or she had read the major theoretical and empirical literature on adolescence. In the mid-1980s there are few, including myself, who would make this same claim because of the radical increase in volumes devoted to adolescence. Although I cease to be personally comforted, I am still professionally disheartened because the increased quantity of output has not been accompanied by a parallel increase in descriptive foundation research that is necessary for a field of study to evolve in a healthy, scientific manner. In this chapter I will review recent proposals for future research agendas for studying adolescence; all essentially ignore this point. In response to them, an alternate research agenda is proposed that argues for an ethological approach to the study of adolescence. This back-to-the-basics agenda is partially fulfilled by the remaining chapters of this manuscript.

Reviewing Research Agendas

The Adolescence of Adolescence Research

During the last two decades there has been more than a simple incremental increase in research on adolescence, and this has been duly noted by a number of recent reviews projecting the future research agenda for the field of adolescence (Berzonsky, 1983; Grinder 1982; Hill, 1982 & 1983; Lerner, 1981). This awakening can be easily documented by counting the number of journal pages that address issues of adolescent development, the journals devoted exclusively to adolescence, the conferences and programs at regional and national meetings that focus on issues of adolescence, funding sources for the study of adolescents (most usually problematic youth), and adolescent textbooks, new and revised, published in recent years (Berzonsky, 1983; Hill, 1982; Lerner,

1981). There is a *Handbook of Adolescent Psychology* (Adelson, 1980), a biennial national conference on adolescence that first met in Tucson in 1982 (Thornburg & Thornburg, 1983), and a Society for Research on Adolescence that was organized in 1984 and met for the first time in March, 1986 at Madison, Wisconsin. Grinder (1982) and Hill (1983) note that the range of topics covered has also grown rapidly as disciplines other than psychology and sociology have contributed to the study of adolescence. Two new books on adolescence illustrate the inter- and multi-disciplinary approach to critical issues of these new scholars of adolescence. Brumberg (in press) focuses on a typically biomedical issue, the fasting of adolescent girls, from a social historical perspective and Hamilton (in preparation) evaluates the cross-cultural educational and work programs for youth of West Germany and the United States.

In his summary of the First Biennial Conference on Adolescent Research, Blyth (1983) reported that many of those present felt that the study of adolescence had moved out of its infancy and childhood and was in its own adolescence, with an appropriate identity crisis:

We are neither true believers in the omnipotence of earlier theorists and researchers nor are we satisfied being rebels who seek simply to disprove the perspectives of previous generations. Rather we are moving beyond these acts of rebellion toward a more complete, complex, and diversified sense of what adolescent development is all about. While we are far from having a mature science of adolescent development, we are moving beyond traditional views toward a new more integrated and testable view. (pp. 157–158)

In some sense the publication of the *Handbook* was a rite of passage (Lerner, 1981), moving the field beyond past theoretical and methodological limitations:

In sum, given the current and potential transitions in the theoretical and methodological approaches to the study of adolescent development, it may be fair to say that the study of adolescence is itself in its adolescence. Although traditional unidisciplinary, often atheoretical, unidirectional, and methodologically univariate and historically insensitive work is still conducted, there is an emergence of new conceptualizations, to be tested by an historically different array of data collection and analysis strategies—these will be used by a cohort of scientists newly concerned with this period for what it can reveal about basic developmental phenomena. (p. 259)

With this explosion of interest and the increase in doctrinaire positions, current researchers employ adolescent subjects not only because of the convenience of such populations, but also because they have a genuine interest in the development of adolescents.

There are, however, additional research responsibilities that must be assumed if the field is to advance beyond its adolescence into its adulthood (Hill, 1983). The research agendas proposed by these writers reflect their best judgment of the future for the study of adolescence.

Many of the issues discussed here have been identified by nearly all reviewers. I limit my consideration of proposals to those that have been presented since 1980.

Longitudinal Research

One of the outstanding contributions to the *Handbook* is the extended chapter by Livson and Peskin (1980), who argue for the continued significance of longitudinal research in studying adolescence. Others (Adams, 1983; Berzonsky, 1983; Blyth, 1983; Hill, 1983; Jorgensen, 1983; Savin-Williams & Demo 1983) agree, placing top priority on this research method for future research on adolescence.

Many note the importance of the early California longitudinal studies. Elder (1980) and Livson and Peskin (1980) have been most vocal in this respect, and yet such studies need replication and expansion. Few have or are willing to undertake such projects, for a variety of reasons that are believed to limit the usefulness and practicality of longitudinal research designs: publication pressures, low short-term payoff, atheoretical perspective, inefficiency, lack of methodolgical rigor, cost. Livson and Peskin (1980) present convincing arguments for the speciousness of these projected limitations and propose, as do Adams (1983) and Berzonsky (1983), shortcuts that include retrospective reports and a variety of seqential—cohort, time, and cross—methods.

Longitudinal studies are essential if adolescence is to be placed within a life course perspective that considers not only the precursors of adolescence and the outcomes of childhood, but also predicts adult development (Lerner, 1981; Livson & Peskin, 1980). Whether one's concern is with the stability of psychological traits over time, such as self-esteem (Savin-Williams & Demo, 1983), or how contextual factors, such as the family, result in changes in psychological states (Hill, 1983), longitudinal research strategies are invaluable.

Despite the myriad problems inherent with the longitudinal perspective, few would disagree with its significance for the future study of adolescence. It will be retrospectively interesting in the near future to pay homage to the brave researchers who overcame the handicaps cited above to study youth within a longitudinal time frame.

Multi-Method, Multi-Trait, Multi-Variate Analysis

Because method variance is usually greater than person variance, single measures and single methods of assessing adolescent personality are extremely suspect (Savin-Williams & Demo, 1983). Past research has relied too heavily on (abused) surveys and questionnaires, which are most useful if employed in conjunction with other, more diverse and personal research strategies, such as participant and non-participant observations, interviews, projective techniques, and other innovative forms (e.g., paging devices to elicit repeated self-report measures used by Csikszentmihalyi & Larson, 1984). Although traditional research approaches may be appropriate for some questions, descriptive, correlational, and ethnographic methods should also be more fully explored (Adams, 1983; Blyth, 1983; Thornburg, 1983). In the classroom ethnographic observation of behavior would complement the abundant educationally based research that has relied almost exclusively on self-report data (Thornburg, 1983).

Hill (1983) argues for a better conceptualization of variables (e.g., "identity") and a more accurate measurement of research dimensions. In addition, Blyth (1983) and Livson and Peskin (1980) advocate an increased use of multivariate techniques of data analysis that allow the data to reveal potentially unexpected relationships, and that permit "the data to reveal whatever threads of predictability do exist, whether or not these threads involve the same or different personality characteristics at the predicting and outcome ages". (Livson & Peskin, 1980: p. 89)

These methodological approaches are mandatory, many of the reviewers maintain, if our future conceptualization and measurement of adolescence are to be multi-dimensional and more accessible to capturing the wholeness and complexity of the lives of adolescents. One-shot, single-measure research strategies produce transient results that have low explanatory power and are unable to further our understanding of adolescence.

Through the Eyes of the Adolescent

Jorgensen (1983) argues for an increased consideration of the phenomenological aspects of adolescent development. In regard to sexuality, the researcher should seek to understand the meaning of sexual development and sexual behavior through the eyes of the adolescent—how she or he experiences sexuality, interprets it, gives it meaning, and acts on it. In other areas, such as emotions, motivations, beliefs, attitudes, and perceptions, future research must sample the adolescent experiences from the world. The adolescent should be asked the meaning of an event, including potentially emotional issues such as puberty (Petersen, Tobin-Richards, & Boxer, 1983).

The Contextual Quality

Future research should continue to clarify the extent and meaning of contextual influences on adolescent development. The individual's personal sense of identity is affected by his or her external existence; several of the reviewers assert that we know far more about the traits of adolescents—their stable, enduring characteristics—than we know about how adolescent behavior is affected by both immediate and historical contexts (Berzonsky, 1983; Blyth, 1983; Hill, 1983). The request is for more socially, ecologically based research that demonstrates how different environmental conditions affect adolescent development (Adams, 1983; Blyth, 1983; Grinder, 1982). Ecological psychologists (Schoggen, 1978) advocate behavioral setting analysis; social psychologists (Bandura, 1978) stress the dynamics of the person-situation interaction.

Peer groups have received the bulk of the attention; familial influences on adolescents need considerably more study (Hill, 1983). Future research must also consider the larger, socio-cultural effects on adolescent behavior (Lerner, 1981). Elder (1980) stresses the historical context; Jorgensen (1983) notes the interface of sociostructural variables such as cultural values on adolescent sexuality; and Thornburg (1983) believes more research should be conducted in schools, especially considering the varieties of inter-school differences (e.g., size).

The influence of Bronfenbrenner's (1979) proposals for the ecology of human development has been and will continue to be felt by the field of adolescene. Whether the context is immediate or historical, reviewers of research agendas have called for increased attention to how the quality of adolescent life is affected by the contexts in which she or he lives. Taken alone, however, this concern is ultimately not sufficient because the adolescent also rebounds and affects the contexts. Livson and Peskin (1980) point out that when we study adolescents and their parents, both the research subject (the adolescent) and the context (parents) have developmental needs that are interwoven. Future research must consider the person, the context, and their interaction.

Intra-Individual Influences

An individual's growth patterns are influenced by parallel and interacting developments occurring simultaneously within the individual. For example, much of the research on pubescence has considered puberty primarily as an independent variable—usually as an event—influencing various aspects of personality and social development of adolescents. In the future, pubescence should also be considered as a dependent, continuous variable that is affected by the individual's physical behavior, such as athletic participation (Hill 1983).

Petersen, Tobin-Richards, and Boxer (1983) note that the direct effect of pubertal processes on cognitive development needs to be explored; Jorgensen (1983) stresses the impact of puberty and its timing on sexual development; and Hill (1983) gives several examples of unresearched areas of intra-individual development: eating and behavior, cognition and social development, and gender role and pubertal development. Perhaps the largest void, according to Hill (1983), is the connection between intra-individual change and social transitions such as movement into high school.

As this section and the preceding one indicate, studying adolescents can no longer be considered to be a simple subject X "direct effects" paradigm. Rather, multiple and complex changes occurring within the individual affect each other and they, in turn, influence and are influenced by contextual processes, transitions, and events occurring on the outside. For example, to study the adolescent-family interaction, it is necessary to consider changes occurring within the adolescent (pubescence, cognition) and each of the parents (generativity and independence needs) as well as larger socio-cultural concerns (attitudes toward family-adolescent conflict). Each of these, in turn, affects the others; for example, a cultural attitude that promotes the norm of conflict within the family may heighten the parents' concern that every slight, normal intra-family conflict is a precursor to delinquency that may, as a result, cause the adolescent to feel increased stress when with the family. So, he or she thus spends more time with peers, learns delinquent activities, rejects the parents and their cultural values, becomes a drug addict, etc.

Life Span

All adolescents have a developmental history, and for most individuals adolescence will eventually become a part of that history. Future research needs to examine childhood precursors of adolescent processes and adult outcomes (Berzonsky, 1983). Developmentalists should study not only short-term effects of their favorite variables, but also the long-term effects of particular events or processes that happen to an adolescent.

Just as early adolescence researchers argued that development does not end in the Freudian childhood, so, too, must future adolescence researchers recognize that development does not end at adolescence (Livson & Peskin, 1980). This life span approach assumes that adolescents are not static beings without a past or a future (Lerner, 1981).

Theory-Research-Application Balance

Perhaps in reaction to the early clinical, psychiatric orientation to the study of adolescence, there has been a tendency among adolescence researchers to become extremely empirical. As a result, much of the research is fragmented with little relevance beyond a limited scope (Thornburg, 1983).

First, there was abundant theory with little empirical research; now, most empirical research is atheoretical (Lerner, 1981). It is not that we need more research, but that we need more theoretically based research (Grinder, 1982). Much of the "theory" that is applied or tested is more conventional wisdom or intuition than sophisticated, systematic theory.

To advance toward a productive future the field must move beyond theoretical and empirical limitations—not so much to repudiate the past as to offer new, interdisciplinary views that encourage a diverse and broad understanding (Blyth, 1983). Popular stereotypes or theories that portray adolescents as society's misfits offer little hope for an increased opportunity to reconceptualize the developments of adolescence.

In a similar manner, no longer can the fields of basic and applied research afford to be divorced from each other. Practitioners must identify their research needs and the researchers must articulate their research interests and interpret their findings to those concerned with theoretical and applied issues (Thornburg, 1983). Both the practitioner and the scientist must, in turn, communicate with the policy makers who have the power to influence the lives of adolescents both directly and indirectly.

Setting a Research Agenda

The research agendas proposed by these reviewers for the study of adolescence offer quite substantial methodological, theoretical, and empirical considerations that are appropriate goals for the study of adolescence, as well as for other times during the life course. The point of departure for this book is its emphasis on two subsets of these concerns: (1) The methodological procedures by which one comes to know the critical and fundamental issues of adolescence and (2) a conceptualization of adolescence that is congruent with an ethological perspective. The former will help to establish a base level of knowledge for the normative occurrence of behavioral phenomena and the latter will offer a theoretical alternative to many of the established explanations of adolescent behavior. In the process of addressing these two issues the research reported here will also underscore the importance of a longitudinal, multi-method and multi-trait research design that is ecologically sensitive to the reality of adolescent life. In noting some of the past methodological and conceptual shortcomings of the field of adolescence, I want to emphasize that in these respects the psychology of adolescence[1] has become in its historical development not unique but a representative subset of not only developmental psychology but also the general field of psychology.

From the experiences of being with adolescents in a variety of contexts and of reading about adolescents in literary, popular, and scientific sources, it is possible to conclude that there are several critical deficiencies in the study of adolescence. Many of these in the theoretical and research literature concerning the nature of adolescence are due primarily to the ways in which social scientists, with a few notable exceptions discussed in Chapter 2, conduct research on youth: relying on self-report of behavior rather than investigating adolescent behavior through observational techniques in the "natural" world of the adolescent—their neighborhoods, schools, families, and recreational activities.

Social scientists also treat adolescents as if youth were removed from the natural order of life. Adolescents are frequently presented as a rare animal with little connection to other species, rather than as continuous in their behavior and ways of constructing their physical and social worlds with their near genetic kin. This omission is certainly not isolated to the study of adolescents; it is only one instance of the more pervasive tendency in developmental psychology to focus on the uniquely human characteristics of our species at the expense of understanding our commonalities within a larger context of the natural world.

Each of these two issues will now be discussed in more detail. Their importance will become increasingly critical in succeeding chapters of this book.

Methodological Issues

My major methodological objections to research on adolescence center on two aspects: its reliance on self-report procedures and on contrived, staged research settings. Others have noted these deficiencies for

---

[1] I limit my critque of research on adolescence to psychological research, not because other disciplines such as sociology and anthropology are immune to the criticisms of the paper, but because of my greater familiarity with the discipline of psychology. In fact, some of the published research on adolesence that best fits my model has been conducted by sociologists and anthropologists emanating from the Chicago School of Sociology community studies. My critique of these studies can be found in Chapter 2.

Psychology in general, which, too quickly, omitted the descriptive stage characteristic of the evolution of other sciences:

It has been said that, in its haste to step into the twentieth century and become a respectable science, Psychology skipped the preliminary descriptive stage that other natural sciences had gone through, and so was soon losing touch with the natural phenomena. (Tinbergen, 1963; p. 411)

Psychology has been predominantly an experimental science ... The descriptive, natural history, ecological phase of science which is so strongly represented in the biological sciences, sociology, anthropology, earth sciences, and astronomy has had virtually no counterpart in psychology. This has left a serious gap in psychological knowledge, for in leaving out ecological methods, psychology has almost completely omitted a basic scientific procedure that is essential if some fundamental problems of human behavior are to be solved. (Barker & Wright, 1955; p. 1)

More recently, Coles (1985a & 1985b) submits the view that Psychology has a tendency to deify theories without first observing and listening, in his case, to children. In a review of these two volumes, Postman (1986) notes that Coles contrasts his observations with the kinds of abstract thinking and tests to "made-up scenarios" practiced by others: "When one listens, he [Coles] believes, theoretical frameworks often seem to lie somewhere between aridness and irrelevancy". (p. 28) His "documentary child psychiatry" is similar in many respects to my advocacy for descriptive studies of adolescents.

Although Hall is generally credited with innovating the scientific study of adolescence (Grinder, 1967), he championed a particular scientific methodology: self-reports. In this regard he reflected the parent discipline, Psychology. The primary emphasis in the study of adolescence has been to understand and discover knowledge solely through the self-reports of adolescent subjects. Who but the individual, after all, is more qualified to make an assessment about one's characteristics? We know far more about what adolescents tell us that they do than what they actually do. The Psychology of Adolescence is currently overwhelmingly the study of perceptions or the perception of behavior and not of behavior as manifested in daily living.[2] Tinbergen (1963) charged that Psychology concentrates on relatively few phenomena and studies them deductively in contrived, staged settings. Psychology moved into the laboratory and other artificial settings before research subjects were observed in their naturalistic settings. This has also been characteristic of the study of adolescence.

---

[2] I am speaking here of the bulk of research on adolescence. There are, fortunately, notable exceptions such as Steinberg's (1981) longitudinal study of adolescent-parent interactions. Although not completely "naturalistic," it approaches what I would like to consider the cutting edge of research on adolescence.

Twenty years ago Bayley (1965) described the current status—both then and now—of the study of adolescence:

When a field of investigation is new, it is necessary to be more exploratory, to make a crude map of the territory in order to get one's bearings, before an exact and detailed map is possible. (p. 186)

In the attempt to be "scientists," developmental psychologists have been far too concerned with controlled, experimental conditions (Livson & Peskin, 1980), forsaking naturalistic research in favor of self-report measures and treatments in clinical, experimental designs. In this regard they are similar to Sommer's (1977) portrait of modern-day social psychologists who have been so preoccupied with maintaining control of their research design that they have confined themselves to contrived encounters and ungeneralizable, uninteresting research findings. In their desire for rigor, developmental psychologists have neglected anthropological field research, perhaps fearing the difficulty of intervening in the ongoing behavior of adolescents in natural contexts where one observes whatever behaviors and events naturally occur or co-occur, and where the interventions of experimental conditions or obtrusive measures necessarily eliminates "naturalness." The sense of controls is alien to naturalistic research. Independent variables that are of interest in terms of affecting a phenomenon under study covary in the natural world, and thus are not truly separable independent factors (Livson & Peskin, 1980). This frightens many who believe that in order to be true scientists they must maintain tight control over their phenomenon. Even when they engage in field research they approach the natural world as if it were an experimental chamber, as a less dank and dark laboratory (Sommer, 1977).

There are those, for example Hartup (1983), who call on their peers to study adolescent behavior in the naturalistic settings in which it occurs. But few have responded, for reasons noted earlier, and because such studies are frequently quite time consuming. Observing behavior over extended periods of time may seem less professionally desirable to the aspiring doctoral or tenure candidate than giving a self-report measure to a class of 500 psychology students that consumes 20 minutes of data collection time. Few dissertation committees would approve "anecdotal observational research" for a thesis; we demand rigor and reliability (Sommer, 1977). Naturalistic settings are more hazardous and less predictable than are controlled or laboratory settings, and self-reports more than the observation of behavior are amenable to simplistic or complex manipulation which can be maneuvered to fulfill the obligations of experimental design.

In particular situations it may be beneficial to introduce a variable artificially into field research (Sommer, 1977). But this short-cut should only be taken if nonreactive data have already been collected and the terrain is familiar. Too many psychologists are quick, however, to assume that their phenomenon cannot be observed directly, thus, apparently supporting the elimination of any observational methodology—contrived or noncontrived.

In a series of studies on one "unobservable" characteristic of adolescents (self-esteem), I discovered that when one subjects such a phenomenon to observational techniques, quite divergent results emerge from those usually reported in the literature (Savin-Williams & Jaquish, 1981). Participant observers and peers may have access to processes not available to the actor (Wells & Marwell, 1976). Individuals are frequently not able to perceive their own personality or behavior apart from situational factors (Jones & Nisbet, 1972). Thus, on the more traditional self-report tasks they may not be sensitive to their overall self-esteem level, but report how they feel at the particular moment when self-regard is assessed. Measures based on others directly observing behavior may be more objective, accurate, informed, and less dependent upon situational cues than are self-report measures (Coombs, 1953). For example, Evert, an adolescent participant in one camp study, was nominated by his 11 peers as highest in self-esteem, popularity, and dominance, and the second most handsome, athletic, and cooperative in his group. Behaviorally, Evert ranked first in altruism and dominance and second in self-esteem. At the close of camp he was awarded the Jack Pine Savage trophy as the outstanding leader and woodsman of his age group. It would not be unreasonable to assume that Evert is an individual with high self-esteem. Yet, on two self-report self-esteem measures, Evert reported a low self-esteem, ranking ninth and eleventh out of 12 boys in his group. Intuitively, I side with the accuracy of the self as presented to others, explaining Evert's reluctance to report high self-esteem as a personality characteristic that may or may not be related to self-esteem.

The "let's-just-take-a-look-and-see" approach advocated by early developmentalists (Bayley, 1965; Jones, 1958) has proved to be beneficial and quite rewarding in a number of instances. For example, in the naturalistic studies of adolescent peer groups to be described in this manuscript, the research design was disrupted several times: One boy entered the study group one week after camp began because of a previous commitment to a hockey camp; a youth was injured and sent home; and an all-camp Bicentennial celebration eliminated collecting data in my five predetermined settings for the day. But these unplanned, natural interruptions became unsought blessings. The first situation gave me the opportunity to observe the behavioral responses of group members when an established group structure is disrupted by the entry of a physically and vocally aggressive individual. One-by-one this new boy systematically disposed of group members, starting with the last ranked boy, and proceeding until he confronted first a draw, and then a defeat at the hands of the second ranked boy. The second situation, removal of an individual from the established group structure, gave information of the opposite sort (those lower in rank each advanced one spot).

Frequently, "accidental findings" can be annoying to the researcher who believes that all "research findings should be deduced from theory and predicted in advance." (Jones, 1958; p. 95) But, Jones asks, do we know enough about development to make all of the relevant predictions? We did not then, and we still do not today:

Our case for reconstructing adolescence implies, of course, a larger viewpoint, to which we now turn: that adolescent personality is no longer to be construed as inherently unchartable, but rather as relatively uncharted. The turmoil and flux of the adolescent condition have too long served as a deterrent to a closer scientific scrutiny on the nature and types of adolescent perturbation and the longitudinal outcomes that they help create and shape. Once these possibilities have been recognized, the longitudinal study of adolescence can be seen as providing a most auspicious field for empirical personality study. It is then that palpable psychophysiological changes and the obvious psychosocial transitions come together to provide, as perhaps at no other time in the formative years, clearly discriminating measurements with a functional and theoretical relevance of what is measured. The potential offered by adolescent longitudinal study for relatively precise naturalistic research in personality-theory construction is just beginning to become apparent; such research is richly possible indeed. (Livson & Peskin, 1980; p. 70)

As noted in the review of research agendas, several (Hill, 1983; Jorgensen, 1983; Thornburg, 1983) have advocated an increased emphasis on naturalistic studies of adolescents. Jorgensen and Thornburg propose to their peers a diversification; conduct fewer experimental and survey/questionnaire studies and more ethnographic research that observes adolescent participants as they interact in natural settings. Jorgensen (1983) emphasized community-based research:

We may be able to answer some of the research questions posed here with greater validity if researchers actually live, work, and play with early adolescents while at the same time observing them and recording data about maturational, psychological, and behavioral changes over a three to five year span. (p. 152)

But this is difficult because human adolescents are not always docile creatures. It is not unusual for an adult to feel inadequate, on guard, and remorseful when in the presence of adolescents. To many developmentalists preschoolers are cuter and less threatening; thus, it is not surprising that most naturalistic studies are conducted with nursery and elementary school age children. Although Hill (1983) places little overall emphasis on the need for naturalistic, observational research, his call for more research on the order of Hollingshead (1949) and Mead (1928) that addresses the experience of adolescents in various social class and ethnic groups can best and, perhaps, only be answered by documenting this experience through naturalistic methodologies. Despite the early, promising observational studies of Hollingshead (1949), Lippitt et al. (1952 & 1959), the Sherifs et al. (1953, 1961, & 1964), Suttles (1968), and Thrasher (1927), this research became an anomaly rather than normative, with a resulting negative consequence for the study of adolescence.[3]

Conceptual Issues

When conducting naturalistic studies of adolescents, developmental psychologists should also recognize an unwanted antagonistic fact: Humans are animals. It appears to be an embarrassment or, if realized, ignored. Certainly, it is underplayed. The "animal nature" of young children, not yet properly socialized, or of adolescents, still enthralled with the trauma of puberty, may be discussed in developmental psychology textbooks, but with humor or with the sense that with proper nurturing "it" will go away. Rarely are our graduate students encouraged to take courses in human genetics, physiology, anatomy, neurology, or psychobiology. When addressed, our biological self is most frequently reserved and packaged for describing the events, seldom the processes, of pubescence.

Not all, however, are so quick to dismiss the interplay of biology with other features of adolescents. For example, Bouchard's "Minnesota Twins" research project has brought together psychologists, psychiatrists, pediatricians, and physiologists to study identical twins reared apart to explore the interdependencies of medical, psychophysiological, psychomotor, emotional, cognitive, personality, and attitudinal aspects of development (Holden, 1980). Kreuz, Rose and Jennings (1972) demonstrated how a psychological factor (stress) can affect the biology (circulating plasma testosterone) of late adolescent military cadets. Udry, Billy, Morris, Groff, and Raj (1985) reported that although socially learned rules inform an adolescent boy when to date and the proper progression of kissing to petting to coitus behavior, male hormones (especially testosterone) determine the *level* of sexual motivation and sexual behavior. Although geneticists, physiologists, and neuro-endocrinologists, through these kinds of studies, have made some progress in influencing the way developmental psychologists think about human nature on a molecular level, disciplines that emphasize a biological perspective on a molar level have had little impact. One such approach is

---

[3] This view is perhaps overdramatized in this paper. Others (e.g., Blyth, personal communication) vehemently disagree, noting that the field of adolescence did not forget these contributions, but built on them, perhaps not as sytematically as would be ideal. I am less inclined to agree, although I recognize this point is debatable.

human ethology, which has a short history as a discipline (Eibl-Eibesfeldt, 1979 & 1985), growing up in the early 1950s and coming of age only recently in terms of textbooks (e.g., Boice, 1983), books of readings (e.g., Omark, Strayer, & Freedman, 1980), and organization (what was to become the International Society of Human Ethology first met in 1974).

The central theoretical position of ethology is that all behavior should be· studied in fundamentally the same manner as other biological phenomena, as part of the adaptive equipment of the organism. Human behavior is on a phylogenetic continuum with that of other animals; we share many fundamental behavior patterns with other primates. Although many behaviors are species-specific and genetically related species may not share a common environmental history due to variations in divergence and convergence (Thompson, 1975), because of a common genetic history species within a particular order have similar reactions to the external world. These commonalities should be studied comparatively to elucidate the evolutionary process (Tinbergen, 1963). But, before these interspecific comparisons are to be made, "What is called for is systematic, species-by-species analysis of *normal behavior patterns*" (Beach, 1978; p. 121). In this regard, researchers of adolescence have much fertile ground for future studies.

Perhaps the early divorce between the biological and social sciences has been beneficial, but now there needs to be a contemporary interaction between the two. Evolutionary biology, ethology, neuro-ethology, and sociobiology have demonstrated their utility in enhancing an increased understanding of human behavior (Masters, 1984). A new volume tentatively titled *Sociobiological Perspectives on Human Development* (MacDonald, in preparation) promises to advance this cause. The observations and research data on nonhuman primates are especially beneficial for developmental psychology:

Neither individual nor collective behavior can be studied adequately from the narrower approach of the anthropocentric psychologist or the historian who focuses exclusively on human accomplishments and failures...The recent expansion of concepts and principles that enliven and challenge the field of developmental psychology stems largely from contributions of ethologists and other behavioral scientists who have taken a broader subject matter than the behavior of any single species. (Riesen, 1974; p. 433)

Thus, human ethology is useful for the study of adolescence because it provides a framework in which to address scientific concerns, both substantive and methodological. If, at birth, an individual enters the present human species, it is at pubescence that he or she becomes a member capable of determining the future of the human species. Although psychologists such as Erikson (1959) consider pubescence to be a critical time in an individual's life course, an ethologist is as concerned with pubescence as a critical time in a species' evolutionary past and future because of its consequences for reproductive maturation, thus making possible the proliferation of the individual's genetic material in succeeding generations, and for gaining independence from the primary caretakers, thus enhancing gene pool diversification (Weisfeld, 1979). Perhaps no other time in the life course is so crucial, to the individual, to his or her society, and to the species.

Weisfeld and Berger (1983) identify universal characteristics of adolescence, features of adolescents across cultures and with parallels (homologies) among primates: pubertal growth spurt, secondary sexual characteristics, intrasexual competition, intergenerational conflict, same-sex aggregation, and interest in infants—with variations between the sexes on these dimensions. Other features are unique to *human* adolescents: the family, play after reaching maturity, continuous sexual receptivity, and menstrual synchrony among others (Weisfeld & Berger, 1983). Several of these themes are further developed within a sociobiological framework by MacDonald (1986).

My concern with these early formulations of an ethological theory of adolescence is similar to my objections with other theories on adolescence: making assertions and reaching conclusions with inadequate data. Although I do not disagree with the content of the ethological perspective, I do not believe that there are sufficient descriptive studies of human adolescents in naturalistic settings to justify more than generating hypotheses concerning the place of adolescence in an evolutionary context. Indeed, we probably know more about the natural behavior of *nonhuman* primate adolescents than we do of human adolescents. This failing is even more urgent in a consideration of the almost total void of naturalistic studies of adolescents in other cultures. Although the morphological and somatic changes of pubescence are well documented, at least within Western populations, knowledge of behavior changes occurring during adolescence is empirically inadequate for the kind of conclusions necessary to support any theoretical framework of adolescent development.

My particular preference for an ethological approach to the study of adolescence is based not so much on its present empirical findings on primate adolescence, but for its potential in terms of methodology, an orientation of describing individual behavior in natural settings, and its theoretical emphases on normal rather than pathological behavior, cross-cultural and cross-species comparisons of behavioral and social patterns, the search for species uniqueness as well as universals, the interplay of the biological organism with its ontogenetic history and its current social context, an integration of different levels of explanation ranging from physiology and genetics to evolutionary theory, and an interest in both developmental change and stability. Chapter 2 presents a further examination of an ethological perspective on human adolescence as it relates to the study of peer relations.

Conclusion

Eventually the research agendas proposed by the post-1980 reviewers of adolescence research may be heeded—or they may never be. The first priority must be to conduct naturalistic, observational studies of adolescents. Other concerns noted by the reviewers are frequently met by ethologically oriented research on adolescence that considers in the research design parameters and effects of the social environment; is longitudinal, albeit short-term; employs other methods, usually some form of peer ratings or self-reports, besides observations of behavior; and looks, if not literally through the eyes of the adolescent, at the world of the adolescent's behavior with an emphasis on reducing interference as much as is possible. If the early social scientists had continued this fundamental, descriptive phase of the study of adolescence, perhaps the research agendas in the 1980s would have appeared less formidable.

It is professionally uncomfortable each year to confront an audience of 200 Ivy League freshman/sophomores in an introductory adolescence course with the statement, "We really know relatively little in regard to how typical adolescents live their typical lives in their typical world. We will spend most of this course dispelling the myths with which you entered this course." I believe ethologically based methodology and theory offer the best hope of correcting the misunderstandings created by our past conceptualizations of adolescence. The initial step in beginning a research agenda for the study of adolescence is to conduct descriptive studies of adolescents in their natural world, employing a variety of observational techniques and theoretical perspectives and sensitizing the research design to include issues that incorporate our species uniqueness and continuity with other animals.

In support of this research agenda, I offer the remaining pages of this volume. Far from complete, the studies described in this book are in the direction in which I feel the future of the study of adolescence should be.

2
An Ethological Perspective on Dominance Behavior

In this chapter I trace the developmental history of my interest in the observational study of adolescent behavior, beginning with my first exposure to sociological and psychological studies of adolescents. I found them unsatisfying. My conversion to an ethological approach to issues of adolescence is then charted, focusing on several basic ethological conceptual and methodological assumptions. Next, questions of human ethology in general and my particular interest in dominance behaviors and relationships among adolescents are presented. These issues form the basis of the succeeding research reported on adolescents of varying ages and of both sexes at summer camp.

Sociological and Social Psychological Studies

As noted in the Preface, I was involved in two seemingly disparate activities during my college undergraduate years: observing the competitive interactions of *Rana pipiens* (leopard frogs) and *clamitans* (green frogs) to *tenebrio* (mealworms) dropped on a flatrock in a glass box (Boice & Williams, 1971; Boice, Quanty, & Williams, 1974) and shepherding groups of adolescents through various summer camps. These two strands were not to come together for some time; first came a diversion, described below, that became a clarifying opportunity for my theoretical and methodological priorities.

Lord of the Flies

In the process of reading literature about adolescents I came across a most compelling account of adolescents in *Lord of the Flies*. In the book, Golding (1955; pp. 6, 7, & 9) describes some of the most subtle and yet effective competitive behaviors among adolescent males recorded by any writer:

He hesitated for a moment, then spoke again, "What's your name?"

The fat boy waited to be asked his name in turn, but this proffer of acquaintance was not made; the fair boy called Ralph smiled vaguely, stood up, and began to make his way once more toward the lagoon. The fat boy hung steadily to his shoulder.

The fat boy glanced over his shoulder, then leaned toward Ralph. He whispered, "They used to call me 'Piggy.'" Ralph shrieked with laughter. He jumped up. "Piggy! Piggy!"

"Ralph—please."

Piggy clasped his hands in apprehension. "I said I didn't want—"

"Piggy! Piggy!"

Ralph danced out into the hot air of the beach and then returned as a fighter-plane, with wings swept back, and machine-gunned Piggy.

"Sche—aa-ow!"

He dived in the sand at Piggy's feet and lay there laughing.

"Piggy!"

Piggy grinned reluctantly, pleased despite himself at even this much recognition.[4]

The occurrence of these kinds of interpersonal interactions are further described by Golding in rather dramatic detail, leading to an exposure of the "animal (beastly, but natural) nature" of adolescent boys.

Social psychological and sociological studies of adolescent males have pursued these themes by investigating the existence of dominance differentiation operating to structure interpersonal group behavior in a manner strikingly reminescent of *Lord of the Flies*. For example, community (Suttles, 1968) and gang (Thrasher, 1927) studies refer to a clearly enuciated and enforced system of power differentiation and patterned regularities within the adolescent reference group. Many of these studies, summarized below, influenced my conception of how best to proceed further.

Thrasher

Thrasher (1927) observed 11- to 17-year old males in Chicago gangs. These ethnic, neighborhood groups varied across most socioeconomic strata, from upper-middle class athletic clubs to lower class tough, criminally oriented gangs.

All groups had a spontaneous social order that was due to internal processes of conflict and competition. This natural inclination for organization was necessary for "corporate behavior and cooperation." The primary structural element was the "two-boy pals"—an intimate relationship between two boys in which one was generally subordinate to the other: "Jerry is running Alfred now."

---

[4] Reprinted by permission of the Putman Publishing Group from *Lord of the Flies* by William Gerald Golding. Copyright (c) 1955 by William Gerald Golding, renewed.

Each boy had a definite status within the group, necessary for leadership and discipline if a more or less harmonious and efficient organization was to accommodate changes in personnel or activity. Three levels of organization permeated most groups: the leader and his lieutenants, the rank and file, and the fringe or hangers-on.

Thrasher noted the importance of the group structure for individual members:

Internally the gang may be viewed as a struggle for recognition ... (an) opportunity to acquire status and hence it plays an essential part in the development of his personality ... It not only defines for him his position in the only society he is greatly concerned with, but it becomes the basis for his conception of himself. (p. 230)

Inevitable conflict within a group served to locate each boy with reference to others. The group structure, according to Thrasher, was an "accommodation of conflicting individualities more or less definitely subordinated and superordinated with reference to each other and the leader." (p. 230) Any standing in the group was better than none; subordinates always had the possibility of improving their status over time.

Thrasher outlined the characteristics of high status individuals, the leaders. All other things being equal, a big, strong boy had a better chance than a "shrimp" for high status. "Natural" differences in physique and aptitudes were important, giving certain individuals advantages. For example, being a bully and possessing athletic ability aided fighting and proved one's masculinity. But, if he were to retain leadership for any length of time, he must be more than a mere bully. Leadership qualities also included gameness, bravery, imagination, experience, and daring— all backed by physical prowess. Most of all, a leader had the ability to make others feel secure in his presence. In making decisions he was quick and firm; he was one of action and of a convincing nature, even when wrong.

Group members seldom verbalized why the leader became the leader; they just knew that he was. Thrasher believed that the gang forms and the leader emerges, rather than a gang forming around a leader.

Finally, Thrasher outlined a number of group roles:

a) Funny Boy: His humor is often an attempt to compensate for some physical disadvantage, such as a high pitched voice.
b) Brains: He is educated, imaginative, and dependable, able to plan things and help the group stay out of trouble by his quick thinking; but, he has little physical force at his disposal.
c) Show-Off: An egotist, bragger, bluffer, and attention seeker, he is one who overestimates himself.
d) Goat: One who is uncommonly dumb and goofy and who always seems to get caught.
e) Sissy: One unwilling to fight, exhibits effeminate traits and cultural pursuits; "Ordinary boys will go to any length to avoid such a role." (p. 234)

Sherifs

Extensive observations have been made by the Sherifs and associates (1953, 1961, 1964) of boys in camp and city settings. Two dozen 10- to 12-year-old boys from a lower-middle class substratum spent 18 days together at a summer camp (Sherif & Sherif, 1953; Sherif et al., 1961). After three days of camp the boys were divided into two equal groups on the basis of camping and athletic skills, physical size, personality, and intelligence; the goal was to splinter initial interpersonal attractions. In all four groups, the staff acted as participant observers; they discerned two well-defined, relatively hierarchical structures in each group on the basis of popularity and social power (leadership or "effective initiative"). The two hierarchies were not the same, even though the most powerful individual was usually the best liked.

In 1964 Sherif directed his attention to more naturally occurring groups of male adolescents. Graduate students went into various socioeconomic settings to observe groups of 6-12 adolescents, ages 15 to 18 years. After several weeks the observers gained an indepth rapport with the group as coach, provider of transportation, etc. Instructed not to write in the presence of the youth, the observers recorded impressions and particular details of behavior for at least 100 observational hours per group. Over time, an observer was able to detect a patterned group structure based on power, control, and sanction of behavior. At first, it was only possible to reliably rank the extreme group members; after several more weeks with the group, the observer deciphered the power rank of the intermediate boys as well.

The alpha individuals employed physical aggression to maintain power, but, as often as not, without any attempt on their part to influence or direct the subordinates' behavior, powerful indivduals were imitated or deferred to by underlings. Shaw, the Red Devil captain (Sherif & Sherif, 1953), was extremely daring, athletic, tough, attractive, intelligent, and popular with peers. He was the captain who enforced his will by threats and physical enocunters. On his birthday, group members were surprised to discover that he was only 12 years old: "I thought you were at least 15!" exclaimed one boy. Crane, the Bull Dog camp leader (Sherif & Sherif, 1953), organized camping trips and softball games; when there was a debate over who should distribute a group prize, group members would only allow Crane to perform this task (cutting a watermelon). He stopped bickering without saying a word; he acted and no one complained.

When group activities changed there was often an alteration in leadership. But, it is interesting to note that a former leader (or perhaps the overall leader who had the most social power) "lets" the other assume leadership. Other social psychologists have substantiated the stability and resistance to change of a group hierarchy based on social power (a term closer to "dominance" than to leadership) (Glidewell, Kantor,

Smith, & Stringer, 1966). Although the leadership structure may vary in accordance with the skills needed for a particular task or activity, the power hierarchy remains constant.

Others

Lippitt, Polansky, and Rosen (1952) used both sociometrics and observations to assess the power dynamics in 32 groups of 11- to 15-year old boys and girls at summer camp. Twenty-four of the groups were for problem or emotionally disturbed adolescents at a specially designed, therapeutic camp. In the other eight groups of seven to nine middle class boys, three observers, on a daily rotating basis, checked behavior from a precategorized observation schedule, recording behavioral contagion (imitation in which the initiator has not communicated intent to evoke the imitated behavior), direct influence attempt (the initiator consciously and deliberately attempts to influence the other to act in a particular manner), involvement in social or nonsocial activities, and "other behavioral indicators" of group status (hostility, affection-seeking, etc.). Sociometrics were given during the first and last weeks to the boys and cabin counselors, asking for an assessment of attributed power ("Who is best at getting the others to do what he wants them to do?"), goodness in sports, best liked, fighting ability, most want to be liked, sex sophistication, and knowledge of campcraft. Additionally, each counselor ranked his group on adult relatedness, impulsiveness, group belongingness need, feeling of acceptance by the group, conformity to group pressures, warmth of relations with peers, social sensitivity, and activity level. The individual listings of the boys on attributed power were highly consensual for the highest and lowest ranks. There was even greater agreement on who ranked in the top and bottom half of the group. This power order was significantly related to the behavioral measures of contagion initiation and successful influence attempts. Individuals seldom used force or physical means to assert their power and yet, there was a significant correlation between camper and counselor ratings of *perceived* fighting ability and attributed power. In the cabin groups of young adolescent boys, attributed power was undifferentiated as to the specific activity or situation:

This is to say, the actor's power may have initially derived from pre-eminence in some particular type of activity or characteristics, e.g., fighting, sports, campcraft, disobeying adults, strength, size, but fellow members tend to generalize this pre-eminence to the general range of group situations and activities. (p. 62)

Although the perception of one's own power in the adolescent male group was significantly related to actual attributed power position, there was a slight tendency for a boy to over- rather than underrank himself. Cabinmates perceived high power individuals as being more skilled in campcraft, personally liked, and frequently identified with than lower status group members; the latter were likely to be either extremely high or low on nonsocial behavior while the former were average. Top-ranked individuals initiated more attempts to influence the behavior of others and, as previously pointed out, to be more successful when so doing. Submissive boys were frequently characterized as withdrawn, queer, bookish, aggressive, hostile, snobbish, and "different." Being a returning camper did not enhance one's power among peers (Lippitt, Polansky, & Rosen, 1952).

Esser (1973) borrowed the "ethological concepts" dominance and territory from Tinbergen and Darwin to study intragroup interactions among 17 emotionally disturbed adolescent boys (ages 9 to 14). For three hours per week for 25 Sunday evenings he observed all "social contact" and "aggressive" behavior. Dominance was equated with aggression (that is, fighting), so his study is of limited value in enlightening the current research. Although the basis is untold, Esser asked cottage parents and staff to rank the boys on "status." JF, who ranked first, was labeled a bully who had little social contact and few total fights; he did not need to fight because others were afraid of him. When he did fight he initiated. The status peck order was not related to "general adjustment" or social contact, but was significantly correlated with initiating fights and territorial fights. Most fights were between closely ranked boys.

In four groups of 11- to 13-year old boys (N = 29) at an athletic oriented summer camp, Koslin, Harrlow, Karlins, and Pargament (1968) observed the Sherifs' "effective initiative" behavior, suggestions offered to and approved by peers. Highly ranked boys were perceived by peers to have high rifle and canoe skills, to be tall, and to perform in tasks of central importance to the group (talk over problems, get things done, spirit leader, helper, sportsman, pal around with, etc.).

A number of other social psychologists have investigated dominance and group structure, referring to a dominant individual as a leader (Glidewell et al., 1966), an egotist (Whiting & Edwards, 1973), a headship (Gibb, 1969) and an authoritarian (Adorno, Frenkel-Brunswik, Levinson, & Stanford, 1950) among others, in large part depending on how dominace is asserted or expressed. One may attempt to exert dominance from various motivational desires: to serve one's own interests, to gain desirable prerequisites, to counter dominate, to humiliate or aggress against another, or to assume leadership over a group (Maccoby & Jacklin, 1974). A dominant person desires power, prestige, and material gain, and manifests ascendance, assertiveness, and social boldness (Gibb, 1969).

My Objections

These studies have a particular sense of truthfulness, based on my experience with groups of adolescents in various naturalistic settings—

camps, church groups, school playgrounds, club meetings, and sport activities. These initial descriptive studies, although intuitively gratifying, were scientifically frustrating. They were faulted for the following reasons: (1) using solely sociometric or nonobservational techniques; (2) not quantifying observational data, but relying on impressionistic accounts; (3) employing contrived groups for artificial purposes or tasks; (4) experimentally manipulating independent variables; and (5) assuming evaluative perspectives of the phenomenon. This last is a major, common drawback. Sherif and Sherif (1964) and Esser (1973) equated dominance behavior with verbal and physical threats and aggression. For some researchers dominance is antiegalitarian and, thus, has negative implications:

In dominance behavior, a person is rigid and inflexible, he has his mind made up; he does not reduce the conflicts of differences by finding a common purpose among differences; rather, he maintains or increases conflict or tension between himself and others, who differ from himself; he expends energy against or in opposition to others. In dominative behavior a person disregards the desires of others, he uses commands, threats, or force to gain his unyielding objectives; he attacks the status of others; he adds to the insecurity of others . . . it is the behavior of an insecure person. (Anderson, 1937; p. 403)

Bales (1970) defines dominance as "upward, negative;" by contrast, leadership is "upward, positive." Leaders have informational, reward, referent, expert, and legitimate power while dominants have coercive and negative power (Collins & Raven, 1969).

This is not to imply that all sociological and social psychological studies fall in all of the above listed "misgivings." Notable exceptions that enlightened my conception of an ideal study include the naturalistic and observational camp, classroom, and neighborhood studies of the Sherifs (1953, 1961, 1964) and Lippitt (Lippitt & Gold, 1959; Lippitt, et al., 1952). Although it is doubtful that Sherif's power hierarchy is an exact replicate of a dominace hierarchy as defined in ethological studies, his research is valuable because of the age group studied, seldom observed in its natural habitat by participant observational techniques. It also appears that Sherif's "captain" is closely analogous to an alpha individual in a dominance hierarchy. Although the traditional social psychological literature is productive in its own right, I felt that I needed to look elsewhere for inspiration, questions, procedures, and interpretations.

Human Ethology

It was during this reading period that I first encountered human ethology, through a graduate course offered by Daniel G. Freedman at the University of Chicago. I will sketch only a minimum of the theoretical and methodological assumptions of human ethology in these pages; for a more thorough review there are human ethology textbooks (e.g., Boice, 1983) and controversy in the pages of *The Behavioral and Brain Sciences* journal (Eibl-Eibesfeldt, 1979). This overview will set the necessary context for a more complete discussion in succeeding chapters of the primary ethological concern of this book–dominance relations among human adolescents.

Defining Ethology

Ethology has its theoretical roots in Darwin (1872), but Lorenz (1935) is considered to be the first to systematically present ethology as a disciplined perspective of behavior. Eibl-Eibesfeldt (1975) defined ethology as "the biology of behavior":

In trying to understand why an animal behaves the way it does, ethologists search for the functions of the observed behavior patterns in order to learn what selection pressures have shaped their evolution. By applying the comparative technique developed in morphology, ethologists attempt to reconstruct the phylogeny of motor patterns. They explore the processes underlying the ontogenetic development and finally search for its causes, investigating the releasing stimuli and the underlying physiological processes. (p. 9-10)

Tinbergen, in his seminal 1963 article "On aims and methods of ethology," outlined the basic components of ethology: the application of a biological, scientific method of study to observable, behavioral phenomena. The four major "problems" of ethology center on the causation, adaptive significance, evolution, and ontogeny of behavior.

In his brief history of ethology, Eibl-Eibensfeldt (1985) noted that ethological concepts and methods are generally accepted by other disciplines. The field has expanded to accommodate the variety of biological inquiries into behavior, from neuro-ethology and brain chemistry with an interest in proximate causes to evolutionary biology and sociobiology with ultimate causation questions. In all cases, however, human behavior is considered to be the result of both programmed phylogenetic adaptations and cultural modifications.

Nonhuman Primate Research

Primatological research reveals to human ethologists the most potentially productive areas and methods for human research. The "message for ethologists," according to Tinbergen (1968), is that the methods rather than the results of primate and animal research should be applied to the study of human behavior. However, results from nonhuman primate research can generate new hypotheses at a fast rate, hypotheses that are probably nearer the mark in explaining real life occurrences than armchair theory (Blurton-Jones, 1972).

This is not to contend that there is *one* primate pattern, but a common thread that runs throughout the primates—phylogenetic unity (Sade, 1981). It is difficult to define with precision what it means to behave as a primate because behavior is dependent on environmental factors, such as ecological niche, population composition and density, and recent group experiences and history, as well as on taxonomic position (Dolhinow, 1972). Thus, the search is not so much for *the* pattern as for a common theme from which variations are derived.

The value of examining developmental issues in species other than our own has been demonstrated through recent reviews of nonhuman primate research on the mother-infant relationship (Swartz & Rosenblum, 1981), paternal behavior (Mitchell & Brandt, 1972; Redican & Taub, 1981), and peer interactions (Rosenblum, Coe, & Bromley, 1975; Savin-Williams, 1980b). In these reviews the adaptive value of various types of associations for children were identified, along with environmental pressures that might account for the diversity of these relations. Similarly, by considering the behavior of nonhuman primate pubescent individuals one gains an understanding of the behavior's evolutionary significance and, thereby, approaches the study of human adolescence with a deepened appreciation of its importance for human growth and development. Knowing the form, content, and function of primate behavior helps to characterize those human behaviors that are more than immediate accommodations to the environment but are built into the very nature of being a primate—whether human or nonhuman.

Medin (1974) suggests that cross-species research is crucial in three respects. First, comparative research elucidates the evolution of behavior: How humans behave now is dependent not only on the immediate situation but, also, on how ancestors faced similar circumstances. Second, such research aids in understanding how the demands of a particular environment have been met by changes in anatomical structures and associated patterns of behavior. And third, cross-species research explicates basic principles and functions of behavioral systems or processes. Thus, in this volume interspecies comparisons within the primate order are frequently made.

I will not argue that humans are necessarily "higher"—or for that matter, "lower"—than other primates; that issue and the relative uniqueness of humans compared to our kin are not of concern here. Although the human capacity for reflection before action enables us to be more complex creatures (McGuinness, 1984), a major task of ethologists is to employ behavioral definitions of the phenomenon under investigation, even if, conceptually, it is usually described with mentalistic characteristics or attributes. An ethologist employs neutral labels to behavior in order to eliminate references to motivational aspects (Bateson, 1968).

The emphasis in this book is to present an ethological perspective of human interaction, not to provide an empirical test of an ethological theory. The nonhuman primate behavior literature was valuable in this regard because it provided a direction in what to observe and when, a model for making sense of the data, and a comparative set of findings to better understand the data I collected. But, as Beach (1978; p. 131) has argued, "The validity of interspecific comparison is limited by the reliability of intraspecific analysis." As noted in Chapter 1 this is not yet possible when comparing human with nonhuman primate behavior because of severe deficiencies on the human side. This volume addresses this shortcoming.

Methodology

In his comparative summary of the basic similarities and differences between ecological psychology and ethology, Schoggen (1978; p. 39) notes, "There is a common dedication to the belief that students of behavior need to correct psychology's deficiency in neglecting the descriptive, natural history phase of scientific development."

Both place a primary importance on observing behavior in the naturalistic settings of ordinary, everyday life. Contrived situations are to be avoided and sampling from the "ongoing stream" of behavior in natural contexts is to be encouraged.

A third similarity is:

In both ecology and ethology, the research method of choice is direct observation by trained observers who rely chiefly upon their perceptive wit and their thorough familiarity with the organism and the main properties of its normal habitat to assure that the observational record is comprehensive and valid. If the problem requires it and circumstances permit, mechanical, photographic, and electronic aids may be employed as supplements to, but rarely as replacements for, the human observer. (Schoggen, 1978; p. 40)

Finally, both distrust "large preselected and untested categories of behavior" (Blurton-Jones, 1972; p. 1) and trust observational procedures that are carefully described and replicated by others (Schoggen, 1978). It is also common for ethologists to rely on data from other species to suggest what categories of behaviors and what interconnections might be fruitful to investigate. I am not sure where ecological psychologists generate the behavior they consider worthy of exploration—unless, of course, they permit the organism to dictate what is observed, which may be everything (for example, *One Boy's Day,* Barker & Wright, 1951).

A major methodological difference between ethology and ecological psychology is the level and focus of attention. Hinde (1966) notes that recorded behavior are of two sorts: molecular, descriptions of what is physically observed, usually involving an analysis of motor patterns, or molar, descriptions of behavior with reference to its consequences. Ecological psychology is a molar science of the environment, frequently focusing on goal-directed or purposive behavior that requires the observer to make low-level inferences about unobservables such as feelings, intentions, and motives. Molecular details are a bonus but are not required (Schoggen, 1978 & personal communication). Ethology follows the biological tradition of being organism-centered, focusing on molecular, observable behavior that may later be combined to define larger concepts. It is at this higher level that inferences may be made (e.g., evolutionary significance of dominance).

Thus, inference is clearly a central part of both approaches to the study of behavior; the difference is that the ecologists encourage the making of inferences during the observational process while the ethologists defer drawing inferences until later in the investigative process. Both approaches have a common ultimate interest in behavior at the molar level but they follow different paths in reaching their objectives. (Schoggen, personal communication)

Ethology frequently addresses questions of the consistency of behavior. Thus, for ethology "development" can imply stability; for many ecological psychologists the research strategy is to center on how individuals change over time and across settings, often to the point of neglecting the vast majority that does not change.

Ethological Perspective of Dominance Interactions

Once exposed to the ethological literature and its primate and nonprimate subsets one cannot ignore the avalanche of papers—theoretical and empirical—on dominance, dominance relationships, and dominance hierarchies. Hinde and Datta (1981) are among many who groan " . . . at the sight of another article on the overused, often misused, overdiscussed but nevertheless often useful concept of dominance." (p. 422) Early papers (Gartlan, 1964; Richards, 1974; Syme, 1974) noted many measurement and conceptual problems; recently these concerns have been summarized by Bernstein (1981) and debated by his colleagues in the pages of *The Behavioral and Brain Sciences* (Volume 4, Number 3, 1981). Although the actors are primarily primatologists, a number of the issues have particular relevance for studies of human primates.

Definition and Measurement

One of the major developments in the literature is a proliferation of definitions of dominance. Critics could easily solicit the methods section of research papers to support their view that the dominance concept ought to be discarded; definitions and measures vary across species, within species, from one lab to another, and from one time to another (Berstein, 1981). Some favor discarding the concept of dominance because it is "... an attempt to describe the product of a number of complex neurobehavioral systems in a single word." (Flannelly & Blanchard, 1981; p. 440) Gartlan (1964, p. 78) agrees:

It is a concept which has probably done much more harm than good and one which has long outlived any usefulness it may once have had; there is no justification for retaining it in an objective behavioral science.

Smuts (1981), however, is not wringing her hands because of the discrepancies; she believes diversity and not harmony is the goal in describing and measuring dominance. More and better hypotheses will then be generated and tested. In particular, one should not expect definitions to be identical for males and females, for all age groups, and for all situations that a species inhabits (Bernstein, 1981; Gage, 1981; Seyfarth, 1981; Smuts, 1981).

In comparative psychology, dominance has traditionally had its reference to such concepts as competition and aggression; one controlling the behavior of another by force or fighting (Schneirla, 1951; Scott, 1953). Wilson (1975) equated dominace and aggression hierarchies: "the set of sustained aggressive-submissive relations among these animals" (p. 279). Thus, dominance interactions are synonymous for many with aggressive or agonistic behavior—fights, threats, displays, supplantations. Although this may be an adequate conception for many species, as the social communicative skills increase among the primates and within a primate's life course, complications emerge and few researchers are so inclined to equate dominance and aggression. They note that a multiplicity of factors other than aggression mediates dominance behavior, including the behavior of the subordinates (supplantation, avoidance, attention) (Bernstein, 1980; Chance, 1967; Rowell, 1974), and that behaviors labeled dominance may serve other functions (e.g., protecting one's kin) (Bernstein, 1981). Because dominance behavior is a subset of all social interactions (Chalmers, 1981; Maxim, 1981), the social skills of the species must be considered when defining what is behavior that dominates. McGuinness (1984) distinguished the two by noting that aggression is the "intention" to harm while dominance is the "intention" to gain control.

This is not to contend that species generality in dominance behavior is impossible to discover (Gage, 1981), or that reliability in various dominance measures within a species is nonexistent (Bernstein, 1981; Smuts, 1981). Gage (1981) argues that the results of empirical inquiry should determine the definition of dominance that an investigator uses; statistical relationships indicate which particular behaviors should be combined to form mega-categories that enhance convenience and validity (Candland & Hoer, 1981).

Dominance Relationships

Dominance *relationships* are inferred and thus not directly observable (Bernstein, 1981). Altmann (1981) argues that they are the inventions of scientists, in the mind and the notebook of the human observer, and are thus important to him or her, and not to the subjects. Dominance relationships are abstractions, a pattern of interindividual relations, and not an activity or attribute of the individual (Bernstein, 1980). Counter to these views, Seyfarth (1981) and Sade (1981) believe many primates recognize intragroup networks and relative dominance ranks. As a theoretical variable, an investigator can infer its existence for particular forms and structures of behavior.

Perhaps the critical factor is the usefulness of the dominance relationship concept in an explanatory sense (Hinde & Datta, 1981). If it allows one to predict with some, although not necessarily perfect, accuracy of who will be dominant and subordinate in a dyadic relationship then, it is a worthy construct to keep (Bernstein, 1981). All dyads are dynamic and, thus, some intransitivity is to be expected. Because of the history of their relationship, both members will learn who is generally the winner and the loser; when the loser voluntarily submits the relationship is recognized. Before this point the relationship was probably a contested one, and may become so in the future.

Hierarchy

The notion of hierarchy is "the principle by which the elements of a whole are ranked in relation to the whole" (Dumont, 1970; p. 66) or, more concisely, "a set of ordered levels" (Whyte, Wilson, & Wilson, 1969; p. vii). Hierarchy thus marks the conceptual integration of the larger and the smaller, and of that which encompasses with that which is encompassed (Dumont, 1970). Hierarchical rank is a societal category—much like age, sex, in-out, normal-abnormal—global in application because it reflects the dilemmas, experiences, and associations that are intrinsic in constructing and maintaining a conceptual framework of the social world.

Pattee (1973) maintains that:

It is a central lesson of biological evolution that increasing complexity of organization is always accompanied by new levels of hierarchical controls. The loss of these controls at any level is usually malignant for the organization under that level. Furthermore, our experience with many different types of complex systems, both natural and artificial, warns us that loss of hierarchical controls often results in sudden catastrophic failure. (p. xi)

The central assumption is that "nature loves hierarchies":

Hierarchical organization is so universal in the biological world that we usually pass it off as the natural way to achieve simplicity or efficiency in a large collection of interacting elements. If asked what the fundamental reason is for hierarchical organization, I suspect most people would simply say, "How else would you do it?". (Pattee, 1973; p. 73)

The empirical observation of hierarchy is well documented, but the explanation of hierarchical structure is more speculative. Most researchers believe that hierarchical structure facilitates the survival of complexity due to its enhancement of integration. By ordering parts in terms of the whole the complexity of the whole is established. Thus, not to see hierarchy, regardless of the level of empirical concern, would be surprising because it would imply chaos.

Dominance Hierarchy

The joining of the two concepts, dominance and hierarchy, has primarily been undertaken by primatologists and ethologists who consider that among social animals with the capability of individual recognition, a dominance hierarchy will be the result of the residual or inevitable inequalities of aptitudes of group members, thus enhancing a "chain of command" (Dumont, 1970). Alcock (1975) asserts that social animals that did not evolve a system of interindividual dominance relations became extinct because "their excess members lived longer during hard times, devoured the countryside, and caused the downfall of the entire group" (p. 229).

The concept of a dominance hierarchy is only useful if it distinguishes group members on other dimensions: "A difference which makes no difference is no difference" (Bernstein, 1981; p. 427). A dominance hierarchy must be shown to be an independent variable influencing dependent variables within the group or that other independent variables affect it across a number of groups (Hinde & Datta, 1981). Multiple groups are necessary to demonstrate that relationships are generalizable and are not due simply to the uniqueness of individual group members. Under the latter conditions is would be difficult to maintain that natural selection was at work (Bernstein, 1981). The correlates should be shown to be biologically important, especially for social roles and patterns of interaction.

Thus, for dominance rank to be an important conceptual tool it must be demonstrated that there are commonalities across groups in characteristics on an Nth ranked individual. But, "We have little evidence that any specific rank causes an individual to behave in a specific fashion, or that a knowledge of numerical ranks allows us to accurately predict the behavior of specific individuals" (Bernstein, 1981; p. 428). Few primatologists have fulfilled this challenge, except in global terms such as top versus bottom or high versus low rankers.

Dominance as a Trait

Bernstein (1981) maintains that dominance is a learned relationship and not an attribute of an individual. One cannot say that one individual has more of a "dominance" trait that another because whether one is dominant or not is dependent on who the other dyadic member is:

Genes lie in the individual and not in the spaces between individuals. Genes influence the absolute and not the relative properties of attributes. Dominance, as a relationship between individuals, is not an absolute property of an individual, but an outcome influenced by multiple properties of individuals. Since dominance must be determined in a social context, it cannot be abstracted as an attribute of an individual. (Bernstein, 1981; p. 422)

Baenninger (1981), however, notes that dominance is not necessarily learned; an individual who routinely wins encounters against both known and unknown others can be said to have more of a dominance trait:

A propensity to initiate spontaneous or competitive encounters in a variety of situations with a variety of opponents could surely reflect some underlying motivational process or trait. (p. 432)

The resolution perhaps lies in the definition of dominance the investigator uses and the reductionistic level at which one defines a trait. Most ethologists would probably agree on some of the attributes of an individual who consistently wins a dyadic dominance contest. Some of these are morphological or biochemical characteristics—for example, physique, physical maturation, glandular activity, adrenocorticotrophin responses (Kaplan, 1981; Sade, 1981)—and others are behaviorally and socially based—for example, aid by kin, past experiences, prior possession of a status (Sade, 1981). Bernstein (1981) emphasizes the learned components, especially the ontogenetic factors of socialization, particular experiences with other group members, and the interaction of experiential and maturational factors. Others such as Maxim (1981) point to biological determinants. His research implicates the importance of the neuronal system in expressing dominance.

The expression and significance of dominance for other social interactions will vary by not only the species, the immediate social conditions, and the "dominance trait" of the dyadic members, but also by other characteristics of the individual such as his or her sex and age (Chalmers, 1981). These two broad categories have been given inadequate attention by primatologists, but are of central concern to human ethologists and researchers of adolescence.

Evolutionary Significance

Although many disagree as to the adaptive significance or fitness of dominance, it is an essential question for ethological investigators. The evolutionary significance of dominance can be examined on a number of bases. For example, the focus can be on the dyadic relationship with an emphasis on the immediate, proximate consequences of being dominant or submissive, or the frame of reference can be on the long-term, ultimate significance of a group dominance hierarchy. In the former, breeding and eating are emphasized (Lott, 1981); in the latter, population regulation, gene flow, and species spread (Kaplan, 1981).

Rowell (1966) concluded that the evolution of dominance hierarchies had a three-dimensional basis: (1) the immediate advantage to the dominant animal such as access to resources, including food, sexual mates, sleeping sites, attention, and locomotor position; (2) the genetic or sexual selection advantage; and (3) the social advantage of group order, peacefulness, and security. Although there is wide disagreement on points of emphasis in these matters, a number of consequences or functions has been attributed to a group dominance hierarchy. Among these are to dissipate intraspecies aggression and overt fighting without negating their useful aspects such as predator protection and population regulation; facilitate known average expectable behavior of individual group members; aid efficiency (less stress) in pursuing personal goals and habitat utilization requiring social mediation; determine commodity acquisition if the supply is limited or the favorability of the habitat declines; structure the limited resources of attention and thus eliminate waste; provide for division of labor and thus aid efficiency; organize activities for an enhancement of group competence and performance; and establish social distance while maintaining sufficient proximity for "groupness" and multisensory familiarity (Bernstein, 1981; Gauthreaux, 1981, Lott, 1981). Poirier (1974) summarizes: "Since each animal knows its position vis-a-vis others and acts accordingly, and as long as each stays in its place, there is minimal disruption" (p. 142).

Competitive behavior is not the only manner in which these objectives or effects can be achieved; maternal behavior can feed and protect and sharing resources among kin can determine who will survive in bad times (Bernstein, 1981). What constitutes an incentive can be unique to an individual, his or her sex or age status, the group, and the species, dependent in part on needs, their experience of the past, and environmental conditions. Becoming dominant itself may be an incentive— seeking prestige (Bernstein, 1981; Itani, 1961; Maxim, 1981).

Wilson (1975) notes that animals who depend for survival on relatively stable group units use dominance rather than territorial behavior to control aggression, adjust mutual relations, and determine priority access to resources: "Dominance behavior is the analog of territorial behavior, differing in that the members of an aggressively organized group of animals coexist within one territory" (p. 279). This does not imply that group living animals do not have territories—their geographic area is compressed into personal space (Hall, 1966) with the center being one's own body rather than a relatively set location.

Less systematic has been the thinking in regard to the benefits or compensations of being subordinate. In a dyadic dominance-submission relationship both must benefit, eventually; this is particularly salient because the submissive member must accept his or her "loss" or recognize his or her subordinate role (Bernstein, 1981). McGuire (1974) suggests that it is adaptive for some individuals to be submissive in order to avoid stress and the fear of real or imagined physical, social, or psychological harm. The potential for stress may be quite high in animals who lack the physical or temperamental equipment—biologically or environmentally induced—to defeat others. Physically losing may have costly consequences, and so, too, may stress. Under stress individuals waste energy, face the prospect of acting "irrationally" or non-adaptively, suffer disease and physical system breakdown (unable to digest food, endocrinolgical imbalances), and are less capable of breeding. For some individuals the costs of competitive interactions may outweigh the benefits of winning (Gauthreaux, 1981).

In other ways being subordinate is advantageous to an individual. One's survival fitness may be considerably higher if submissive behavior is displayed than if one were to make an all-out effort to dislodge the most dominant group member. Alexander (1974) notes that like other group members a subordinate individual is informed by the various group dyadic interactions "when and how to display aggression, and when and how to withhold and appease and withdraw" (p. 330). With such knowledge one increases his or her survival and reproductive chances by remaining in the group. In many social species individuals face little hope of survival if alone, and are almost universally excluded from breeding (Wilson, 1975). But, a submissive group male will probably survive, eating with the group and benefiting from predator protection, with the outside chance of occasional breeding opportunities. By staying with the group, a subordinate individual may also enhance his or her inclusive fitness by aiding the survival opportunities of closely related kin. Furthermore, in most instances the dominance ordering is not rigid because top ranking individuals migrate or die; thus, by staying with the group as a subordinate or peripheral member, one has a chance to advance in dominance status.

Bernstein (1981) argues that evolutionary pressures act on attributes of the individuals involved in the encounter and not on the dominance relationship itself:

... organizational structure and rankings are an outcome of the relative influences of attribute expressions among all the members of the group at any one time and, as such, are only indirectly subject to selection. Social organization is selected for only to the extent that individual traits produce the organization and are selected for in the individuals. (p. 424)

Those attributes include memories, learning abilities, social skills, and physical traits; attributes which are not just for dominance. In fact, they probably evolved for other purposes and now function as adaptive because they enhanced the selective pressures for those very attributes which permit their expression (Bernstein, 1981). If, however, dominance relationships have little biological meaning beyond the dyad, then perhaps it is not worth pursuing the evolutionary significance of dominance (Banks, 1981).

These speculations, however, have been the result of soul searching rather than the result of experimentation and systematic observation (Sade, 1981). These most difficult questions are also the most difficult to answer; thus, I save them for the final chapter of this book.

Humans

Ethologists such as Lorenz (1966) and Tinbergen (1968) argued that humans, congruent with other primates, genetically harbor a number of behavioral propensities that on a group level has the net effect of establishing a system of status differentiation that is necessary for group formation and maintenance (Rowell, 1966). Thus, humans are predisposed to form hierarchical dominance relations when engaged in interpersonal behavior within the context of a social group. The alternative to "fitting in" is to become peripheralized to the group, as a solitaire, or as a member of a "bachelor group," or to leave one's natal group for another. The data for female human or even nonhuman primates have not yet been sufficiently collected to allow for many generalizations (Small, 1984). Although not explicitly stated, the predisposition to establish stable dominance relations does not appear to be solely male conceived. It is "human nature" to create hierarchical orders based on dominance and submission behaviors:

The nub of the historical argument is that during the formative periods of human anatomy and bodily structure—which are broadly replicated in today's model of the human—patterns of social differentiation in the dominance form were also developing, and it is this prior phenomenon which governs the occurrence of dominance hierarchies in contemporary societies, rather than only a variety of formed or historical circumstances. (Tiger, 1970; p. 295)

Present Research

In 1932 the primatologist Zuckerman asserted that an adequate primate sociology is not possible without reference to the principle of dominance.

During a lecture at the University of Chicago 45 years later, ornithologist Marler made the same point: "It would be disastrous to discard the concept of dominance to explain group interactions."

Can one conclude the same when describing the internal structure and interactions of adolescent groups? This issue is explored through a series of descriptive studies of dominance and submission behaviors and hierarchies in groups of male and female adolescents. Four major questions are addressed:

1. Can a social system be described in terms of dyadic dominance and submission behaviors?
2. If so, how stable is this group structure over time and across behavior settings? Is dominance a trait, an attribute of the individual or a state, dependent on the context in which it occurs?
3. What are the physical, psychological, and social characteristics of those who occupy the various status positions?
4. Are the answers to the above questions different for adolescent groups of various ages and for girls as opposed to boys?

In addition, it is of interest to speculate as to the functions such a group structure have for individuals (individual selection) and for the group (group selection). In this quest both objective and impressionistic sources of data will be used.

The present series of studies focuses on social interactions of adolescents in naturalistic settings. Only observable behavior is recorded, with little reference to the organism's feelings, motivations, or psychological processes. Issues of both stability and change are addressed; the center stays with the individual and not the environment. Categories of behavior were generated from studies of both human and nonhuman primates and issues examined bear much similarity with those of other ethologists studying nonhuman animals reviewed in this chapter. The definition of dominance employed here is congruent with the ethological perspective that emphasizes a holistic approach and incongruent with social psychological research that compartmentalizes leadership, influence, power, authority, and dominance, and that frequently equates dominance with aggression.

Chapter 3 describes the setting, participating youth, and research methods. The data are presented, first in an impressionistic account in Chapter 4 and Chapter 5, and then in a more quantified form in Chapter 6. Extensions of the dominance research on early adolescents are presented in Chapter 7 (middle to late adolescence), Chapter 8 (adolescent altruism), and Chapter 9 (trait conceptualizations of dominance and altruism). Chapter 10 summarizes and editorializes the results and implications of the research reported in this book.

3
Camp Wancaooah

In this chapter the primary context for the research reported in this book, Camp Wancaooah, is presented in some detail. The camp setting as well as the youths who participated in the project are described, replacing the actual names with fictitious ones based on their final group dominance status.[1] What constituted meaningful data, how and when data were collected, and data analysis techniques are also described to provide the reader with a comprehensive view of the research methodology.

Setting

The setting is two sex-segregated, adjacent summer camps in the North Central United States. Privately owned and financed, Camp Wancaooah has a 65-year legacy of developing character, citizenship, and leadership in young Americans. The program emphasizes:

... opportunities for leadership development, balanced activity, friendly competition, the acceptance of responsibility for oneself and the groups in which one lives, and the development of close relationships with leaders in which the deeper personal concerns of life can be confronted and meaningfully discussed. (Leaders' Handbook, p. 1)

Historically and programmatically the organization operating the camps is similar to the Boy/Girl Scouts and the YMCA/YWCA. A Boys Camp and a Girls Camp are on the same parcel of land, but separated by sand dunes, a forest, and a mythical barbwire fence.

Camp Wancaooah has over 400 acres of natural forests, sand dunes, and lakes, encouraging such recreational and interest activities as

---

[1] If the name begins with the letter "a" (for alpha), then the individual (e.g., Andy, Ann) was most dominant in his or her group; with a "b" (beta), second; with a "g" (gamma), third; with a "d" (delta), fourth; with an "e" (epsilon), fifth; and with an "o" (omega), last.

overnight camping, water sports, athletic activities, and wood and leather crafts. Summertime temperatures are usually moderate in the heavily wooded center of the camps where the single room cabins are located. On the two waterfronts—a small inlet lake and one of the Great Lakes—a suntan can be carefully but easily nurtured.

The campers, over 200 in Boys Camp and nearly 300 in Girls Camp, range in age from 10 to 17 years and are divided into four age units with 8 to 12 age-homogeneous cabin groups, led by a college-age cabin counselor. For the five weeks of camp each cabin group follows a daily schedule, nearly identical for both camps, as follows:

Girls Camp

A. Morning
    7:15 Wake Up—Cabin Clean Up
    8:00 Opening Ceremonies—Exercises
    8:15 Breakfast
    9:30 Christian Ideals Discussion
    10:00 First Interest Group Period
    11:00 Second Interest Group Period
    12:00 Mini-Interest Group Period
B. Afternoon
    12:45 Lunch
    1:30 All-Camp Assembly
    2:30 Rest Hour
    3:45 Athletic Games
    5:00 Free Swim or Time
C. Evening
    6:00 Supper
    7:15 Vespers
    8:15 Nights Doings (Activities)
    10:00 Lights Out

Boys Camp

A. Morning
    8:15 Wake Up
    8:45 Breakfast
    9:15 Cabin Clean Up
    10:00 Christian Ideals
          Discussion
    10:30 First Interest Group/
          Athletic Game Period
    11:45 Second Interest Group/
          Athletic Game Period
    12:50 All-Camp Assembly
B. Afternoon
    1:15 Lunch
    2:00 Rest Hour
    3:00 Instructional Swim
    4:00 Cabin Time
C. Evening
    6:00 Supper
    6:30 Free Time
    7:30 Vespers
    8:15 Nights Doings (Activities)
    10:15 Lights Out

The camp schedule is structured but also flexible: Between most periods or events is a 10 to 30 minute "free time" that can be spent with the cabin group, other friends, or alone and on "special days" and Sundays the schedule is frequently altered or loosely organized. Swimming, canoeing, sailing, and other waterfront activities are included in the interest group periods. The cabin group is together for an average of 13 to 18 hours per 24 hour time period.

Participating Youth

Over the course of five summers 10 of these cabin groups, six male and four female, were extensively observed for the five week camp session. The 31 male and 20 female adolescents were from upper-middle class

Group No.	Number	Sex	Age	Publication
1	6	male	12–13	Savin-Williams, 1976, 1979 & 1980a
2	6	male	12–14	Savin-Williams, 1979 & 1980a
3	4	male	11–12	Savin-Williams, 1979
4	4	male	12–13	Savin-Williams, 1979
5	5	female	12–13	Savin-Williams, 1979 & 1980b
6	5	female	13–14	Savin-Williams, 1979 & 1980b
7	5	female	12–13	Savin-Williams, 1979 & 1980b
8	5	female	12–13	Savin-Williams, 1979 & 1980b
9	6	male	15–17	Savin-Williams, 1980c
10	5	male	14–16	Savin-Williams, 1980c

suburban or small city families who could afford to send their child to summer camp. A limited number of scholarships allowed other youths, primarily minority, to attend. The youths were for the most part mentally, physically, and emotionally healthy individuals from intact white, protestant families. Seven (14%) of the youths are minority group members (Black, Native American, Asian), eight (16%) are Catholic, and 12 (24%) are from a one-parent or separated home. All but 14 (27%) had been to the camp during previous summers.

The youths were randomly assigned before entry to their cabin group by the camp administration, following a policy of diversity in geographic representation and athletic ability, similarity in age, and not placing returning campers in cabin groups with friends. Significant exceptions were occasionally made to this last policy.

The 11 youths in cabins Nine and Ten were counselors-in-training (CITs) for the summer; they substituted for cabin counselors on days off. Selection for the program, based on demonstrated or potential leadership ability was not highly competitive as two of every three applicants were accepted. Data collection procedures and assessments from these two groups are discussed separately at the close of this chapter.

Pilot Study

In developing a definition of dominance for this study I reviewed both the ethological and the social psychological (especially play behavior) literatures summarized in Chapter 2. Twenty-one behavioral indices of dominance and submission were delineated as observable with a group of adolescents at summer camp (Savin-Willams & Freedman, 1977). These were tested with a group of six 12 and 13 year old boys at Camp Wancaooah the summer before the start of the primary study (Savin-Williams, 1977). Using Gellert's (1961) scheme, the 21 were reduced to 12 indices after data collection by consolidating and combining seldom observed events into more broadly defined categories. For example, "verbal threats" and "physical assertiveness without contact" formed "verbal/physical threats"; "takes object away" and "physical supplant-ation" formed the new category "physical or object displacement." The categories used in this pilot study were further refined by delineating specific subcategories of behavior and labeling them as overt or indirect. This latter procedure made possible a means of analyzing the data across the various indices of dominance and submission on a new dimension: overtness or indirectness. The advantages of these broader mega-categories—ease of observing and recording, training other observers, reliability measures—have been noted by others (Jay & Elliott, 1984); refinements may not necessarily increase validity and they usually decrease reliability.

In the pilot study specific behaviors, regardless of the consequences of the act, were recorded as indicative of dominance status. Strayer (1980) identified this as the "second approach" in describing dominance:

... it attempts to identify a set of behavioral patterns which can provide an empirical and ecologically valid basis for the evaluation of individual differences in social status. This research strategy involves demonstrating that certain behavioral patterns in the social repertoire share important characteristics, and thus can be regrouped into more comprehensive, descriptive categories. (p. 445)

This functional approach is a common one in primate studies and, as noted in Chapter 2, has been criticized by Bernstein (1980 & 1981) because dominance is a relationship term and is thus dependent on an outcome.

This problem was avoided by separating the functional question from the descriptive one in the other study groups. The concern in recording data was not on the motivational, causal, or "why" aspects of behavior, which cannot be observed (Bernstein, 1980). Rather, observations were based on the occurrence of particular types of behavior that *resulted* in a particular consequence: one individual asserting power over or being given power by another individual—Strayer's (1980) third approach.

In this book I use dominance as an eclectic term referring to specific varieties of behavior occurring in a dyad in which one pair member asserts or expresses power and/or authority over the other. In the process influence may have preceded and leadership in a group may result. Aggression may or may not be behaviorally involved. In fact, as the frequency of aggressive behavior decreases after early childhood, it is a necessity to define dominance in a non-physical, non-aggressive fashion during adolescence (Weisfeld & Weisfeld, 1984). Dominance can be used to describe a person ("a dominant individual") or to indicate a social role or position ("the most dominant in the group") without reference to responsibilities or obligations. This usage is incongruent, in part, with Bernstein (1980 & 1981) because although I accept his contention that dominance is expressed only in social contexts, I also believe that as a higher, hypothetical term dominance is also an attribute of an individual. The evidence and the constellation of the *dominance trait* will be explored further in Chapter 9.

Thus, an important issue in considering the dominance group structure is a point made some time ago by Chapple (1940): Hierarchies depend on the ability of one group member to evoke a proper response from another. This point was reiterated by Rowell (1974), who emphasized the submissive act as a necessary component of the dominance encounter. Unfortunately, few human studies (see Savin-Williams & Freedman, 1977) adequately record the various patterns of behavior that connote a subordinate status postion. It is necessary to examine not only the behavior of group members when they initiate dominance but also the response of the subordinates who may initiate their own subordination by recognizing the dominance status of cabinmates. Perhaps it is the behavior of subordinates, who give their attention to other group members, that allows a group hierarchy to be formed and maintained (Bernstein, 1980; Chance, 1967).

A concept that has a number of behavioral component parts becomes a powerful tool in analysis. Many of the most interesting findings of the present research were made possible by such a multi-factorial approach, for example, sex and status position differences in styles of exerting dominance and submission. It also provided the necessary data to answer the question if frequency of occurrence and accuracy of prediciton are always identical relationships.

Procedures

Observational Data

The four female and two male counselors who were participant observers of cabin groups One through Eight recorded from the first to the last day of camp—excluding most Sundays and their personal days off—all verbal and physical dominance interactions occurring between two group members when the entire group was together. Using the event sampling technique, "all occurrences of some behaviors" (Altmann, 1974), observations were systematically dispersed throughout the daily schedule during five behavior settings: rising from and going to bed (bedtimes), meals, cabin clean up-rest hour, cabin discussions, and activities. Observations consumed an average of slightly less than three hours per day per cabin (total hours observed, 692).

At the time of the study three of the female counselors—Joyce, Carol, and Debby—were University of Chicago graduate students; the other, Cathy, was a University of Chicago undergraduate. Prior to their observations all had had extensive camp experiences as campers and as counselors. I observed three of the male cabins, one each during three summers while at the Univeristy of Chicago. Tom, a Dension University undergraduate, was employed one summer to record his cabin activities.

The focus was on the dynamics of social interactions within dyads—the outcome of dominance oriented interactions—and not on the individual differences approach that pays attention only to frequency of occurrence of dominance behavior (Strayer, 1980). Thus, if A ordered B to pick up his clothes and he obeyed, then the interaction was recorded as, "A over B, direct order." If, however, B replied "Eat 'em!" and refused to obey, then the interaction was, "B over A, counter dominance." This interaction could conceivably become a verbal argument, with the individual having the last word registered as the dominant one. If C entered into the encounter, saying, for example, after the first A-B exchange, "Yeah, B, pick up your damn clothes," then only dyadic dominance interactions would be recorded (that is: "A over B, direct order"; "C over B, direct order"; and "A over C, imitation"—assuming that B complied to both requests).

Dominance and submission were categorized according to the following indices of behavior, derived from observations of primatologists, social psychologists, and human ethologists and pretested in the pilot study (Savin-Williams, 1977) (X accorded dominance over Y in each instance). Subcategories with "*" indicate overt forms; the remainder are classified as indirect.

1. *Verbal directive:* X verbally communicates to Y what to do and Y complies.
   *a. direct order or request
   b. indirect directive or suggestion of behavior
   c. giving unsolicited advice or information
2. *Verbal ridicule:* X raises his/her status or lowers Y's by verbally abusing Y or by putting himself or herself in a good light at the expense of Y. Y does not contradict, usually withdrawing from further interaction.
   *a. name calling or teasing through direct confrontation
   b. talk about; verbal put down; gossip or cattiness through a third person
   *c. bragging or boastful behavior
3. *Physical assertiveness with contact:* X pushes, shoves, kicks, or hits Y. Y assumes a submissive posture, flees, or, if asserts self in turn, loses.
   *a. overt aggressiveness—in earnest
   *b. play fighting—in fun and with a smile
4. *Recognition:* Y acts in such a way as to place X in a more powerful position. X becomes a social monitor for Y.
   a. imitating or modeling behavior, appearance, or speech; agree with

   b.   ask for approval of behavior or appearance; apologize
   c.   give compliments or favors; ask where is; defend
   d.   ask or solicit information or advice; divulge information; wait
       for
5. *Physical or object displacement:* X takes an object away from Y, or X
   approaches Y and Y moves away
  *a.   direct removal or supplantation
  *b.   not asking to borrow; moving into space; maintaining a privileged
       position
6. *Verbal or physical threat:* X asserts verbal or physical authority over Y,
   who does not counter.
  *a.   verbal challenge, usually with threat of bodily harm
  *b.   physical challenge without making actual physical contact;
       glaring
7. *Counter dominance:* X, commanded by Y, assertively or passively
   disobeys and Y does not pursue the demand.
  *a.   ignoring a direct order or request
   b.   ignoring the other; shunning; spatial exclusion
8. *Verbal control:* X verbally argues or battles with Y and has the last
   word, or monopolizes the content and structure of the verbal
   interaction.
  *a.   arguments or battles; direct refutation
   b.   monopolizes a conversation; interrupts the other's speech
   c.   contradictions without anger; corrections

Analysis of Observational Data

Dominance behavior occurring in all possible dyadic combinations of
individuals in a cabin group was segmented by indice, setting, and time.
Within each dyad behavior was examined separately for each of the eight
indices of dominance. For each indice a group hierarchy was constructed
(see method below) and these eight rank orders were then compared. In
all groups the individuals ranked significanctly the same across the eight
indices; correlations ranged from .45 to .79, all significant to the .05 level.
Thus, these eight categories of dominance were aggregated to form the
overall behavioral definition of dominance and submission that is used
throughout this book.

In a similar fashion, the data for all dyads in a group were compared
for each of the five settings in which behavior was recorded. In all groups
individuals ranked significantly the same regardless of the setting in
which their interactions occurred; correlations ranged from .66 to .91, all
significant to the .01 level. Thus, setting patterns are seldom discussed in
the text because there were few variations.

To allow for a more detailed analysis of the data and to gain a sense of
longitudinal development over the camp session in each cabin, the

observational data were divided into three time periods for each cabin group. These three time periods correspond to three temporal thirds of camp, usually 10 days each. Cabin members were rank-ordered for each time period in the same manner as described below, summing indices and settings. Significant changes occurred during the camp session, and these are described in succeeding chapters.

Dominance hierarchy. A group dominance structure was constructed by summing the dyadic interactions, regardless of indice, setting, and time. A dominance relationship between two individuals existed only if in subsequent encounters there was a significant probability that the same individual would be most dominant. The number one position was given to the cabin member with the highest number of cabinmates significantly dominated in pair-wise interactions; the number two position, to the next highest number; and so forth. In case of ties, an individual was placed higher if he or she dominated the fellow tie-maker more than the reverse and if he or she had a higher overall dominance success percentage.

Reversal rate and group stability. The reversal rate, or transgressions against the dominance hierarchy (and thus was calculated *post hoc*), is the percentage of the total number of dominance behaviors occurring within a group in which the Ys dominate the Xs, by time period and by the entirety of the camp session. Stability is defined as the significance level of the reversal rate; if the reversal rate was significantly (.05) less than hierarchical congruent behavior (Xs dominate Ys) then the group during a particular time period or the camp session was said to be "stable."

Reliability Checks

Precamp. Before camp the four female counselors-to-be and I observed volleyball and softball games of junior high school students at the University of Chicago Laboratory School. I spent two to three hours with each of the women pointing out and categorizing instances of dominance behavior. Precamp reliability checks were then conducted during softball games. The correlations between each of the women and me were only moderate, ranging from .47 to .62. When specific category was eliminated from the analysis then the correlations increased by an average of 10 points.

Camp. During the second week of camp Debby and Joyce exchanged cabin groups for the lunch meal (45 minutes). Eighty-three percent of the dyadic interactions recorded were in agreement with the other's five week dyadic dominance data.

During the third week the other male counselor, Tom, and I exchanged cabin groups for the lunch meal; a week later we traded groups for an entire day. Despite the disruption in the ongoing cabin life of having a new counselor for a day, the data indicate little variation between the two of us in the relative dominance status of the boys, overtness levels, per hour frequencies of dominance behavior, reversal rates, primary categories of behavior utilized, and overall dominance success of the individual boys.[2]

Postcamp. Joyce, Carol, Debby, and I coded a five minute tape recording of a cabin discussion of the pilot study group of boys, accompanied by a written transcript, for indices of dominance behavior. Reliability correlations among the four of us ranged from .71 to .89; variations stemmed from my tendency to record a slightly higher number of indirect dyadic interactions. Most discrepancies among the four of us were of omission rather than of kind; that is, when we observed dominance behavior we agreed on its indice type.

Sociometric Placings

Even though the traditional ethological method advocates directly recording the behavior of individuals as it occurs and deemphasizes

---

[2] Tom's per hour frequency of observed dominance behavior in my (SW) cabin was somewhat lower than the five week average recorded by me (16.0 vs. 19.3), but not different from the previous days' average (18.0 and 16.0). Because 90% of the behavior recorded by Tom in his one day with Cabin Four involved one boy, Andy, as a participant, it is not possible to construct a dominance hierarchy from his data. Andy was, however, the most dominant, successful 83% of the time (SW: 71%) as he significantly dominated all other boys in the cabin. When asked at the end of the day to rank order the group on dominance behavior, Tom's ranking was identical to the overall behavioral dominance hierarchy. His reversal rate (20%) was lower than my 34%. Seventy-five percent of the recorded behavior was overt (SW: 88%); 60% was ridicule, directive, and verbal control behaviors (SW: 54%). Tom did not, however, observe nearly the level (5%) of physical assertiveness that I did (21%).

I observed a frequency of dominance behavior occurring in Tom's cabin that was slightly higher than his overall average (25.4 vs. 19.3), but not greater than the preceding day's 30.0 average. According to my observations Alex was the most dominant boy in Cabin Three with a success rate of 89% (Tom: 91%), significantly dominating all cabinmates. Guy was the number two individual for both observers (SW: 42%; Tom: 46%). It was difficult to distinguish the dominance status of the other boys in both data bases. The reversal rate that I recorded (22%) was almost identical to the overall reversal rate (21%). According to my data the four boys of Cabin Three ranked significantly the same on the eight indices and five settings. Verbal directives (SW: 8%; Tom: 11%) and rest hour-clean up behavior (SW: 22%; Tom: 14%) were the best predictors of dominance status. My independent assessment of the intelligence, physical attractiveness, and leadership of Cabin Three boys correlated perfectly with Tom's orderings.

Thus, the inevitable differences between the two of us in leadership style, personal behaviors, and observation techniques apparently did not alter the basic dominance patterns of dyadic relationships among the cabin boys.

indirect measures such as questionnaires and ratings scales (McGrew, 1972; Omark, 1980), to implement a diversified, holistic approach in methodology and a potential validity check for the observational data the direct observations were supplemented with measures that use our species' linguistic specialization (Blurton-Jones, 1982). This is Strayer's (1980) first approach to assessing dominance status and by its incorporation the classical mind/body dualism is reduced (Omark, 1980). Dominance and various other sociometrics were given to the adolescents; not all measures were completed by each group, at their discretion (cabin groups completing the placements are indicated in parentheses):

a) *Dominance rankings.* During the first (all cabins) and last (One, Two, Four, Six) weeks of camp each individual was asked to "List the campers in the cabin, including yourself, in order of toughness or dominance." A similar questionnaire (all) was given to junior counselors after they assumed leadership over a cabin on the counselor's day off.

b) *Leadership traits.* After the first dominance ranking campers were asked (all but One) to write the qualities that an ideal leader should have, to reach a group consensus on these characteristics, and to rank each other on the inculcation of the traits.

c) *Friendship rankings.* During the first (all but Five) and last (One, Two, Four, Six) weeks of camp, one day after the dominance sociometric was given, each participant was asked to "List in order your friends in the group." As in all sociometrics, results were not known to the cabin counselor or to the youth (left to the discretion of the cabin counselor) until the camp session was over.

d) *Friendship traits.* Immediately after the completion of the first friendship sociometric individuals were asked (Three, Four, Six, Seven, Eight) to write the qualities that an ideal friend should have and to reach a consensus on those traits.

e) *Adjective characterization exercise.* Midway through camp each cabin member was instructed (One, Two, Three, Four, Six) to write the name of the one cabin member, including himself or herself "Who is the _____ in the cabin." Forty adjectives or roles were verbally inserted in the blank by the cabin counselor:

1. shortest
2. funniest
3. weakest (strength)
4. most religious
5. tallest
6. least intelligent
7. bully
8. brown-noser (counselor's pet)
9. quietest
10. most athletic
11. heaviest
12. most liked by the counse
13. smiler
14. ugliest
15. friendliest
16. best little chief
17. most feminine
18. strongest

19. most mature	30. loudest
20. leader	31. lightest
21. worst little chief	32. most serious
22. smartest	33. most dominant
23. prettiest/most handsome	34. least liked by the
24. richest	counselor
25. poorest	35. most immature
26. least religious	36. most masculine
27. most creative	37. most popular
28. follower	38. most submissive
29. least liked by the group	39. most stubborn
	40. dolt (awkward, does
	stupid things)

These were given in random order.

f) *Athletic assessment.* Cabin members were asked (One, Two, Three, Four) to rank each other on athletic ability for each sport played at camp. These were then averaged for an overall athletic ranking.

These sociometrics were given either during a time set aside by the camp program for cabin discussion on topics conducive "to get to know oneself and the group in which one lives" or during rest hour.

Tests, Measurements, and Observations

To discover the physical, behavioral, and social attributes that characterize the various dominance status positions within a group, several tests, measurements, and observations were conducted during the five weeks of camp.

a) *Body surface assessment* (all cabins): body mass was derived by multiplying weight × height × a constant (Gallagher & Brouha, 1943).
b) *Pubertal development* (all): based on pubic hair, breast, and genitalia development (Tanner, 1962).
c) *Overtness* (all): the percentage of the total number of dominance behaviors that was overt (see indices of dominance behavior).
d) *Socioempathy* (all): the accuracy in rank-ordering the cabin group on the dominance sociometric.
e) *Socioeconomic status* (all): based on Hollingshead's index of socioeconomic status of occupations of the primary "breadwinner."
f) *Bed position* (all): the distance in inches from each camper's bed to the cabin counselor's bed, with the closest being the number one position.
g) *Individual and family characteristics* (all): from the camper and parent application forms information was gleaned in terms of the youth's

chronological age, race, religion, and year at camp; the family situation (separated, divorced, stable, etc.); number and age of siblings; geographical location; and parental comments on their offspring.

h) *Physical attractiveness* (all): as evaluated by the cabin counselor.

i) *Counselor's favorites* (all): each counselor ranked her or his group relative to how well she or he liked each of them.

j) *Intelligence* (all): assessed by the cabin counselor or by the general information, similarities, and digit span sub-tests of the WISC (1965) for an estimation of intelligence (One, Two).

k) *Athletic ability* (Five, Six, Seven, Eight): assessed by the counselor based on observations of the campers.

l) *Leadership* (One, Two Four): from the observational record, the percentage of times an individual's suggestion for group activities was accepted by the group.

m) *Hiking position* (One, Two, Four): the predominant position of individuals as the group hiked single-file on various occasions.

n) *Sit beside* (Five, Eight): whenever group members had free choice (non-assigned) of sitting position it was noted who sat by whom.

o) *Physical fitness* (One, Two): assessed by the Harvard Step Test that considers the speed by which pulse rate recovers to its normal level following exercise.

p) *Creativity* (One, Two): assessed by the Torrance Test of Creativity (Torrance, 1966); important are the elements fluency, flexibility, originality, and elaboration in the usage of words and ideas.

There was little agreement[3] among the four dimensions that the counselor was asked to rank order his or her cabin group—physical attractiveness, athletic ability, intelligence, and counselor's favorites. Thus, a cabin counselor was apparently using different criteria when he or she rank ordered group members on the four traits.

Cabin Groups Nine and Ten

Five days per week each of the CIT groups ate breakfast together, cleaned the cabin, and met briefly to discuss the coming day before assuming the role of junior counselor in a cabin of boys. The group came together at the end of the day to discuss experiences, share stories, and relax during free time. During the other two days the boys had free time and engaged in recreation activities, rest, and reading or went as a group for a day off away from the camp grounds.

---

[3] Ws ranged from .23 to .65 with the last being the only significant one, $p < .05$ (Kendall Coefficient of Concordance; Siegel, 1956). "W" is a measure of the relation among rankings of individuals.

The same indices of dominance behavior used in the early adolescents groups measured dominance in the two CIT groups. As program director for the two groups of counselors-in-training, I daily recorded all occurrences of dominance encounters between group members during three behavior settings for a total of 77 hours. Unobstrusive recording of observations was conducted immediately after breakfast interactions (30 minutes per day), during cabin discussions by "taking minutes" (30 minutes per day), and during free time while writing letters or program notes (45 minutes per day).

During the last week of the camp session the boys were instructed to rank group members, including self, on the following factors: (1) dominance, (2) outcamping skills, (3) athletic ability, (4) creativity, (5) intelligence, (6) crafts skill, (7) friendship, (8) cabin spirit, and (9) best cabin leader. These exercises were conducted as part of the group assessment project and thus were not construed as being unusual or unexpected.

A number of other assessments were made during the camp session to note their relationship with the behavioral dominance hierarchy. These are similar to the measures previously described: chronological age, pubertal maturation, socioeconomic status, physical size, hiking position, bed position, overtness, and frequency of involvement in dominance interactions.

Human Subjects

Based on previous studies of adolescents in natural settings (Polansky et al., 1949; Sherif et al., 1953, 1961, 1964), I decided not to inform the youth before data were collected that they were participants in the study. The assumption was not that such information would discredit the study's results, but that it would infringe on and complicate the observer's primary role as cabin counselor (see the Polansky et al., 1949 situation).

Prior to the observations the camp administration was informed of and gave consent to the study. Parents of the campers had in the process of registering their child for camp signed over to the camp a "physical and moral" release form. The University of Chicago and Cornell University human subjects committees approved the research design with the stipulation that all future reports of the data be such that individual camper names not be identified.

We informed our cabin group at the close of camp, in language appropriate to the youth's level of understanding, the methodology, motives, and purposes of the research project. No camper expressed objection to nor suspicion of being observed. Occasionally, a camper noted that his or her cabin counselor was writing a lot, usually in the form, "You sure write a lot of letters." A vague answer sufficed to defray the curiosity.

Detailed recording of dyadic behavior by the cabin counselor was feasible because the youth believed he or she was engaged in normal counselor activities. For example, during athletic games the counselor was keeping score; during cabin meetings, taking minutes; and during clean up-rest hour, writing letters. When instantaneous recording was not possible (mealtimes), the interactions were recorded immediately afterwards. The effect that the observer as a group member may have had on the study's results is unknown; every attempt was made within reason for the physical and psychological safety of the adolescents to adopt a laissez-faire attitude during cabin dominance encounters. The detailed behavioral recordings, the enriching data examples, and the existence of the study itself would not have been possible if a dual cabin counselor/observer role had not been assumed.

In the next two chapters the natural history of each cabin group is chronologically described, focusing on both impressionistic and numerical data.

4
Life in the Male Cabin Groups

Cabin One

Overview

Cabin power was primarily controlled by one boy and his sidekick. They felt stuck with a "nurdish" cabin consisting of an oversized goon, two losers, and a whimpy follower. When asked by the cabin counselor (SW) what would make cabin life more pleasant, they replied: "There's no way to end the conflict except to change personalities." There were times when the constant complaining and criticizing occurring in Cabin One became difficult for everyone to bear. Never forming a compatible cabin group, the boys could not complete a cooperative squares game. One would finish his square and then laugh at the others, not realizing that he had to rearrange his pieces in order for the group to succeed.

It was a spirited, active, and camp-wide reknowned group. A sense of responsibility and sensitivity toward others became more prevalent during the last week of camp.

The Camp Session

By the first night of camp Alan commanded cabin power and respect. During the traditional first night dirty joke time, Alan's sordid tales were the only ones thought humorous by all. Earlier in the evening cabinmates wanted to construct bunk beds, but Alan said that he would not sleep in one; none were made. After the first athletic game Gary accused him of trying to be a hero; Alan responded in a manner that soon became his trademark: "So what! What does it matter?" Alan could only be foiled if the entire cabin "got on his case," as when he refused to be quiet one evening until the other five in unison shouted, "Shut up!" By the next morning, he was again resisting group pressure. It was his turn to be the cabin cruiser, but he refused to return for more syrup and pancakes, despite the urging of Gary and Ed, because, "I've had all I want." Even though Gary then called Alan a dirty name, he said it so softly that Alan could easily ignore it.

Bobby also told first night dirty jokes, long after everyone else had had enough. He was quick to interrupt others' jokes with "Hey, I've got another one!" Although Bobby remembered Alan from the previous summer, they were not friends before camp began. But within hours after arrival they were inseparable; dyadic interactions between them were the most frequent in the cabin. Together they played tennis, 4-square, and basketball, and after several meals they invented "groin juice"—mixing together all of the liquid garbage (milk, ketchup, soup de jour, bug juice, etc.). When one served or cleaned the table the other helped. Gary said on Day 5 that he wanted to trade Alan to another cabin, keeping Bobby; Alan replied, "If one of us goes then both go." Bobby chimed agreement.

The pair enjoyed the position of experienced and knowledgeable returning campers, making camp life difficult and unpleasant for the other four Cabin One boys. They ridiculed them for being "doltish" because they did not know what to do. The brunt of the ridicule was distributed to a different Cabin One member during the course of the camp session. First, it was Don who was remembered and disliked from last summer. Then, they turned on Oscar when he arrived on Day 4. After the middle of camp Ed knew little relief from the pair's tongue lashing.

Much of the name calling and hostility centered on homosexual themes: fag, mo, and groin were favorite names to call each other. Don frequently made "obscene" comments that centered on homosexuality, male anatomy, and various "deviant" acts. Alan was initially upset when he discovered that Don would be in Cabin One. They had several fights during the first week of camp, provoked in most instances by Alan. For example, one day the boys sprayed Cutters bug repellant into a biffy (restroom) wall hole while Don was using the facilities. Don bantered with them, enjoying the attention; suddenly he explosively bolted out of the biffy and attacked Alan, the instigator of the bug spray fogging, scratching him with his long fingernails before being pinned in a headlock. Several days later, Alan was throwing hard boiled eggs at a tree when one accidentally hit Don who was coming up the path by the tree. Don again exploded, running, screaming, and swinging wildly. In both cases, after a period of silence, Alan and Bobby looked at each other and laughed, ridiculing Don's sissy fighting style. Alan and Don soon established a mode of co-existence that made life together possible for the remaining four weeks. After the first third of camp their frequency of dyadic dominance fell 50%; their frequency of physical assertions, 90%.

Alan and Bobby chastized Oscar for his lack of athletic abilities within hours after his arrival on Day 4: "Boy, are you bad! You can't even hit the ball like a boy, girl!" At lunch Oscar sat in "Bobby's chair." Alan shouted, "Get up! That's Bobby's chair, you dolt! Do you hear Oscar! Get out NOW!" Bobby refused to pass food to Oscar until the latter said "please", and when the chocolate cake came, Alan and Bobby made sure that Oscar received the last, and hence, the smallest piece. After lunch Bobby excluded Oscar from the decision making process in planning next week's activities by replying "What a waste!" to every idea that Oscar suggested. On the afternoon hike, the pair unmercifully ridiculed him in regard to the slowness of his hiking pace, his poor athletic ability, his sissy clothes, etc. Several times Oscar retaliated, but it only increased the verbal abuse. He finally walked at the rear of the hiking progression, talking with Don.

Thus, Oscar quickly learned his place, falling immediately after arrival to the lower echelons of cabin prestige and power. He coped with his unenviable environment by withdrawing from or complying with most potentially threatening encounters. When Alan demanded that he get seconds for lunch, Oscar pointed out that it was not his but Bobby's turn to be the table cruiser. Alan replied, "Allright, you'll have to face the consequences!" Without asking what those consequences might be, Oscar brought the extra potato chips. That afternoon Bobby told Oscar to turn off his radio. Oscar "compromised" by turning the radio down; but 30 seconds later he jumped out of bed and turned the radio off, saying to on one in particular, "I don't want to listen to that talking."

Over the camp session Oscar seldom engaged in dominance en-counters with Alan and Bobby; he was moderately successful during counter dominance interactions. Otherwise, both Alan and Bobby dominated him at a highly consistent rate.

Even though it was Gary's first summer at camp he was familiar with the camp grounds, program, and purpose (other family members attended the camp in the past). Rather than explore the grounds the first few days as most first year campers did, Gary spent his free time in the cabin reading comic books. Within several days Gary began his infamous "manhandling" behavior: grabbing a cabinmate and lifting and shaking him. This was relatively easy due to his physical size advantage and advanced pubertal maturation. During one rest hour time Alan took him to task for his boast of having the largest penis (two card lengths the boys later reported). His threats were seldom taken seriously by either Gary or the victim. But, they soon became a source of irritation; his cabinmates resented his superior strength, and, at times, Gary hurt them. On Day 5 he accidentally grabbed Ed too hard, hurting him and ripping his shirt. Alan and Bobby's defense against Gary's macho behavior was to say he was trying to rape them.

The animosity between Alan and Gary was especially intense. Despite the fact that Gary was five inches taller and 40 pounds heavier, Alan dominated him in 90% of their physical assertive encounters. For example, on Day 10 Gary spit out the cabin, accidentally hitting Alan who was picking up trash. Alan ran into the cabin and hit Gary, who lay cowering in his sleeping bag. As camp progressed, Gary became more subservient to Alan, primarily by obeying his verbal directives and by recognition behaviors. By the last third of camp Alan was dominant in over 90% of their dominance encounters.

Perhaps because Bobby was 10 inches shorter and 60 pounds lighter than Gary, he did not fare well against him in physical interactions. His verbal behavior, however, kept him dominant; although Gary dominated Bobby during physical threats and assertiveness encounters, Bobby was the more dominant in over 90% of their verbal ridicule interactions. Bobby's verbal harrassment ceased only when Gary offered to buy him a Coke in return for an end to the "homo" names. It worked; their level of dominance interactions declined by two-thirds as camp progressed.

The only cabinmate that Alan and Bobby responded to positively during the first third of camp was Ed. The first week Ed was extremely shy, seldom speaking except in a soft and halting manner. To the others he was the "baby"; they claimed that he should have been placed in the next youngest age unit. They were amused the first night when he asked what a prostitute was.

During the first week of camp Alan and Bobby "adopted" Ed, almost as a kid brother. Ed accepted this role, for by it he gained recognition, acceptance, and status. But, he overplayed the role; everywhere Alan and Bobby went Ed was sure to go. He imitated their speech patterns, calling for a "penis butter and jelly" sandwich. When Bobby nominated Don as the "cabin fag", Ed quickly agreed. Ed soon earned the nickname, "the shadow." Being with the two most dominant boys in the cabin buffered Ed against the condemnations of Don and Oscar and the physical manhandling of Gary. When Ed made the last out during a softball game, cabin ridicule stopped only when Alan said, "He's still the best player in the cabin!" On Day 5 Gary teased Ed for his physical and social immaturity. Ed was silent until Alan and Bobby defended him; then he, too, verbally abused Gary. Alan and Bobby also led Ed into trouble; when SW found Alan and Ed skipping the all-camp assembly the second day of camp, it was clear that although Alan knew he was guilty, Ed did not.

The state of dominance relations in Cabin One was most explicit during an acorn fight occurring during the end of the first third of camp. Two battles formed: (1) Alan, Bobby and Ed versus Gary and (2) Don versus Oscar. Alan and Bobby soon separated to create their own battle; Alan was the victor, chasing Bobby and, eventually, accidentally hurting him. Without the support of Alan and Bobby, Ed ran for the tree, chased and hit by Gary. The second battle was won by Oscar; Don did not refute his victory claim. All then chased Don, throwing acorns. Thus, the fight revealed: Alan-Bobby-Ed over Gary; Alan over Bobby; Gary over Ed; Oscar over Don; and the group over Don. The Time One behavioral dominance hierarchy listed, in order: Alan, Bobby, Gary, Ed, Oscar and Don—a duplicate of the acorn fight results.

Alan and Bobby were not pleased to be "stuck" with their cabinmates. Several times during the first weeks of camp they arranged the lunch table so that they were on one side, and the other four sat crowded on the other. During a cabin discussion Bobby asked Alan, "Who don't you like?" Alan replied, "Gary, Don, and Oscar." Bobby agreed.

The two were also the keenest of competitors. After four days of camp SW wrote in his notebook:

Bobby and Alan are the dominant forces in the cabin, but I cannot tell who is the most dominant of the two. Perhaps it is a coalition. They are good friends, and competitors, spending a lot of time together away from the rest.

They called each other "homo" names, grabbed belongings from the other, asked where the other was, ordered the other to come do something, and refused to answer or wait for the other. The second day of camp the boys were hiking on the sand dunes when Alan failed to follow Bobby's lead at a fork in the path. Gary and Ed followed him and Don followed Bobby. Later, at the cabin, the two argued at to which path was faster. On Day 4 Bobby told Alan to play 4-square with him. Alan said that he did not want to and so Bobby left, only to return several minutes later. This time he asked Alan to come; Alan refused and Bobby called him a "lazy groin." Bobby left, returned, and ordered Alan to go with him. Alan agreed, "As soon as I spray Cutters on my legs." Bobby tried to hurry him, "My dead groin could do it faster," and then left. Alan yelled, "Wait! You mo!" Bobby did not and Alan stayed in the cabin.

Dominance relations between the two were clarified as camp progressed. Their Day 9 play fight almost became serious; five days later Alan forced Bobby to beg for a comic book, physically pushed him out of a chair in the eating lodge, refused to play tennis until Bobby asked for a third time, and grabbed the weekly activity planning sheet away from him. The two were of equal status in ridicule and recognition behaviors, but Alan was clearly superior in displacements and physical assertiveness. The pair had almost five times as many counter dominance interactions than might be expected by chance. By the last third of camp Alan was dominating Bobby in four of every five dominance encounters, an increase of over 20 percentage points from Time One. The two were perceived by the group on Day 24 dominance sociometric, however, as being of equal rank.

Alan's power and authority increased as camp progressed. His success percentage rose 11 points from the first to the last third of camp. He also became more popular, moving from third to most popular on the last week friendship sociometric. Alan flaunted his superior dominance status as he rose in power. When the group reminded him after the second week of camp that he had lost enough inspection points to receive a "peanut butter grundy" (peanut butter place in the underwear), Alan responded, "And just who is going to do it?!" No one volunteered. Several days later during lunch he announced that he did not want his dessert. Gary yelled, "I want it!" Seizing the opportunity, Alan demanded that Gary say "Please"; Gary obliged. He had Gary beg on his knees and roll over on the floor in the dining hall. Alan laughed as Gary ate his dessert.

Alan, with Bobby's help, also used his power to disrupt Ed's camping experience. When the cabin group hiked on the afternoon of Day 8, Alan and Bobby, as was their custom, ran far ahead. Ed attempted to tag along, much to the consternation of the pair. Jokingly, Alan nicknamed Ed "the shadow." During lunch the next day, Alan decided to give Ed a hard time clearing and cleaning the table, demanding seconds and "accidentally" squirting ketchup on the table. Bobby readily joined the fun, yelling "Get busy cruiser!" That evening while being chased by Alan and Bobby—they were going to give him a peanut butter grundy for not being a good table cruiser—Ed stubbed his toe, sending him to the health clinic. Afterward SW found Ed crying, but rather than condemn his "friends," he praised them for being nice to him, even though he admitted that at times they gave him a hard time.

Although Alan was prepared to end this harassment after the stubbed toe incident, Bobby continued the battle. He ridiculed Ed for being so dirty, which was in part justified because Ed seldom showered, and he wore the same swimming trunks as underwear the entire camp session; more than anyone else in the cabin, he won the mealtime "dirty face and hand" award. But Bobby went to extremes: setting up a physical barrier between him and Ed at the lunch table, throwing his "stinking Adidas" shoes out of the cabin, and nicknaming Ed "the health hazard." Although Alan's involvment with Ed decreased in frequency as camp progressed, the opposite was true between Bobby and Ed. By the last third of camp Ed was completely subordinated by Bobby as their level of interaction became the third highest in the cabin. Ed dominated either Alan or Bobby in only seven of 121 directive and riducule encounters.

The other three cabin members were more than willing to "step on" Ed while he was down. Despite the fact that the overall frequency rate was decreasing, Ed received an inordinate barrage of agonistic behavior from cabinmates. Alan and Bobby quadrupled the number of times they dominanted him during the second seven days in comparison to the first seven days of camp. Not to be outdone, the two boys below Ed in the dominance hierarchy (Oscar and Don) quintupled their dominance over him during the same period. The net effect was to lower Ed to last place and to raise Don and Oscar one notch. Time Two was the period of camp when Ed's frequency of dominance interactions increased 22 percentage points and his dominance success percentage fell 22 points.

Although Oscar dominated Ed during Time Two, Ed was more dominant during both the first and last thirds of camp. During the third week Ed was "playing" the piano in the eating lodge when Oscar demanded that he be allowed to play some "real" music. Ed refused even after Oscar attempted to physically remove him from the piano bench. Ed freed himself and began pounding again.

Through the first third of camp Don was subordinate to the other boys in Cabin One. For example, on Day 3 Ed asked him if he could use his bug spray; after finishing, Alan and then Bobby used it, emptying it to one half of its former contents. Initially Don's filthy language and jokes were amusing, but the others tired of them, demanding that he grow up.

As camp progressed, Don became more withdrawn and less subservient. He talked back and resisted directives, especially in serving seconds at mealtimes when it was not his turn. The last week he screamed "Go to hell!" in the eating lodge after the others demanded that he interrupt his dinner to get seconds. The behavior of Ed and Oscar especially irritated Don. He once told Ed to shut up or he would slit his throat. On Day 15 he grabbed Oscar's letter and threw it outside the cabin. Oscar demanded that Don retrieve it, which he did not. Two days later Oscar accidentally knocked Don's elbow during lunch. He responded by taking a vicious swing at Oscar and shoving his soup bowl off the table.

Oscar dominated Don during the first two time periods, primarily through verbal directives, but by the last third of camp Don was clearly the more dominant of the two. During this time the level of interactions between the two tripled its Time Two and quadrupled its Time One rate. This new power was achieved primarily as the result of Don countering and refusing Oscar's demands.

The same pattern was also true in regard to Don's behavior with Ed. The two were mutual "least best friends." During the middle of camp Don exerted his prominence over Ed, the time when the level of interactions between the two was twice the expected level. For the camp period the dyad was the second most frequently interacting competitors, especially during verbal ridicule encounters when Don was most dominant over Ed; during physical assertiveness the reverse occurred: Ed dominated Don.

Don thus moved from the omega to the delta position as camp progressed. During Time One his 16% dominance success rate was the lowest in Cabin One; during the last third of camp his percentage, 53%, was the second highest in the cabin. On the dominance sociometrics he moved from last to third.

Gary and Don were best friends, yet Gary dominanted Don in 100% of their dominance encounters during his rise to prominence the last third of camp. The two seldom interacted; however, the number of threat behaviors between the two—usually in fun and jest—was the highest for any dyad. Gary was dominant in all of these. On the other hand, the two were never observed arguing.

While Don's status rose during the last third of camp, Oscar's was on the downs. For example, Oscar dominated Ed during the middle of camp, but Ed returned to his Time One dominance over Oscar during the last weeks of camp. After unmercifully ridiculing Oscar immediately after his arrival, Alan and Bobby essentially left him alone. Oscar selected Alan as his best friend on Day 12, a reversal of his Day 4 selection. But during the last week of camp Alan defended Ed against Oscar's verbal attacks, turning on Oscar with a barrage of directives and name calling as he and Bobby dominated Oscar in 33 of 34 such encounters. Oscar's dominance success fell from near 50% to 10%, tumbling him from the delta to the omega position.

It was during this time when Ed moved from his Time Two low dominance success percentage and omega postion to exerting dominance over Oscar and frequently Gary.

By the end of camp Alan had solidified, almost cemented, his most dominant position in Cabin One. Although Bobby was a threat during the first weeks of camp, by the third week Alan was convincingly dominating him. As Alan's friendship with Bobby eroded, Alan renewed his friendship with Ed, with the resulting rise in Ed's status in the cabin. Meanwhile, Don had clearly established himself as the most prominent among the three lowest ranked boys.

The Data

Ridicule was the most common form of dominance behavior observed, more than the combined total of the second (directives) and third (counter dominance) most frequently observed; threats and displacements were seldom observed, together representing only 7% of the total. Eighty-three percent of the behavior was overt in form.

From Time One to Time Two there was a slight decrease in the per hour occurrence of dominance behavior; but the Time Three frequency was 50% lower than the Time One level. There was considerable variance in the daily frequency averages. Five days, all occurring within the first two weeks of camp, were exceptionally high, coinciding with the entrance of Oscar into the group, the Alan-Don fight, the acorn fight, and the putdown of Ed. Dominance encounters were most likely to occur during cabin discussions and least so during mealtimes.

Of the 15 dyads in Cabin One, 12 were significant in directionality. The three exceptions involved the lowest ranked individuals. During the first third of camp the order after Alan, Bobby, and Gary was Ed, Oscar, and Don. During Time Two Ed slipped into the omega slot and the other two moved up a notch. It was Oscar's turn to drop to the sixth postion during Time Three with Don and Ed moving up one place. Seven of these nine time period pairings among the three were statistically significant; the other two approached significance.

It was during Time Three that the reversal rate fell seven points to a highly significant 18%. Still, during the "unsettled" first two thirds of camp, the percentage of transgressions against the dominance hierarchy was significantly less than hierarchical harmonious behavior.

On both Day 3 and Day 24, the boys' individual rankings of cabinmates on dominance were significantly intercorrelated and were in agreement with the behavioral dominance hierarchy of Time One and Time Three, respectively. During the first and last weeks of camp a junior counselor stayed with Cabin One on SW's day off. When asked the following day for an assessment of the cabin dominance rank order, their listings correlated significantly with the behavioral hierarchy.

The six boys ranked significantly the same regardless of the indice or the behavior setting. Verbal directives was the best predictor of the overall dominance hierarchy; during counter dominance behaviors subordinates were most likely to dominate high ranking members. Alan and Bobby ranked one-two in all five settings.

Only two dimensions significantly differentiated the six boys on dominance status: closeness of bed position and leadership. Dominance rank was also highly correlated with active involvement in dominance encounters, athletic ability, hiking order, physical fitness, chronological age, and middle camp popularity.

There was a strong tendency for individuals to interact most with those closest to them on the dominance hierarchy. There was little relationship between bed position and friendship and between friendship and dominance rank as both Ed and Oscar chose Alan as their best friend. Three boys overranked themselves on the dominance sociometric; the other three were either accurate or underranked themselves.

Conclusions

In most aspects of camp life, Alan's presence was felt. He organized and directed athletic games, telling who to play where and for how long. During the all-camp capture the flag game, counter to Gary's desire to be on the suicide offensive squad, Alan told Gary to play defense—to protect the flag, usually a most unexciting position. Even though Alan was not the tribal chief and, thus, had no legitimate authority to tell Gary where to play, Gary accepted this directive as fact. Alan also assumed leadership on hikes, being in the first two positions 86% of the time and inititating group movement after rest stops. After one such stop on Day 4, Gary told the group, "Well, it's time to move." No one moved. Alan left and Bobby shouted, "Wait up!" The rest followed.

Together, Bobby and Alan practically dictated the cabin activities for each week. Seventy-seven percent of the activities nominated that were approved by the group were suggested by either Alan or Bobby. When others did not initially agree with their ideas, Alan and Bobby exerted sufficient non-physical pressure to change their votes. If someone suggested an idea that they did not like, it was summarily dismissed with "What a waste!" When the group planned their carnival booth for the all-camp fair, individuals did not express their wishes until hearing Alan's and Bobby's opinions. Even after the decision, Bobby elected to set up his own booth, which helped the cabin win the first place prize.

Other, more informal activities were "failures" unless they had the support of Alan and Bobby. For example, Gary, Don, and Oscar wanted to punish Ed for being so dirty by giving him a peanut butter grundy. But, they were not willing to initiate the act until Alan and Bobby, who were reading comics at the time, agreed to help them.

Alan and Bobby seemed to have special privileges in the eyes of cabinmates. For example, Alan called Gary a "perverted groin" and no response was given. But, when Don called him the same name, Gary threatened, "I'm gonna bash your head down so you've gotta untie your shoes to sneeze." And, at dinner one evening Ed chose to pass the dessert to Bobby rather than to Don, even though Don was closer to him.

Alan and Bobby frequently assumed the role and duties of the cabin counselor. Bobby collected money from cabinmates for horseback riding. Alan conducted the cabin "horse 'n goggles," a random process game by which extra food, usually desserts, were distributed. Most cabins only entrusted their cabin counselor to be impartial in this activity. Indeed, several times during camp Alan challenged SW's authority. For example, during Bobby's "fag of the cabin" contest on Day 18, SW jokingly suggested, "Alan and Bobby." Gary quickly seconded, and Don and Oscar chimed "Yeah!" Not to be so easily subordinated, Alan invented a new category, "Leader fag." With this nomination, he again gained the support of the Cabin One boys.

The other group members were also vital to group functioning. For example, even though Alan and Bobby dictated the theme of the carnival booths, the others, especially Oscar, did the necessary work of constructing the booths. Once the cabin flag design was approved by Alan it was Oscar, "because you're so creative," who made and painted the flag. Gary was occasionally the peace keeper, using his physical size to separate Alan and Don during their fight and to defend underdogs under harassment from Alan and Bobby. Gary was willing to change beds with Ed until he remembered that it would place him next to Bobby: "He'd not like it if I was so close to him. No use to cause problems."

Despite the manner in which Alan and Bobby treated the other Cabin One boys, they were the two most popular boys in the cabin. With Alan and Bobby, cabin life was always exciting and spirited, if not comforting.

Cabin Two

Overview

Despite the first five days of rain, the boys in Cabin Two were quite compatible. There were no major conflicts or problems—almost immediate group cohesion—as two boys working together had almost complete control of cabin power and authority.

This compatibility was shaken when a sixth group member arrived one week late. An individual accustomed to exerting himself aggressively and frequently, he temporarily disrupted the cabin's power structure. All adjusted, including the latecomer, and group cohesion was characteristic of the remaining weeks of camp.

The Camp Session

Ara walked into the cabin on Day 1, selected the bed closest to SW, and immediately instructed several other boys where to place their trunks. That evening Ara suggested progressive story telling, until they "got sleepy." After Bjorn and Doug told short, "dirty" segments, Ara began his story of "Billy Jack-Off" and "John-Man"; three times he emphasized the masculinity of his hero. As his story appeared to have no end, the others grew impatient. Bjorn and Doug suggested several times that he "might be" extending his contribution. When Ernie and Omar were finally allowed to contribute, no one laughed, and they were cut short by Bjorn's "Next!" Doug's plots were the weirdest, twisting strange facets of fantasy, comic book reality, and school life. But, it was Ara's deviations that provoked the most laughter.

The next morning Ara and Bjorn refuted Omar's statements concerning events occurring last summer. Later that day Ara initiated a game whereby he chased and 'handkerchief whipped" cabinmates; when Omar refused to play he was ostracized by the others. Thus, by the end of two days the boys were behaving "as if" they recognized status differentiation among themselves. On the Day 3 dominance sociometric, they unanimously agreed that Ara was the most dominant and that Ernie and Omar were the most subordinate.

During the first five days of camp it rained. Forced to spend much initial time together, the nature of power relations was evident and enforced. During a Day 3 thunderstorm, Ara was cheating during a poker game. Omar said several times that his luck could not be so bad, but he did not accuse Ara of cheating. When SW later asked Ara about his behavior, his reply was straightforward: "If he's not smart enough to catch me, then he gets what's comin' to him." Two days later when Ara was not cheating, and losing, he said, "I'm bored" and threw down his cards, thus thwarting the spectacle of losing to Omar.

At the first cabin meeting, no idea for cabin activities was passed that Ara or Bjorn did not support (suggest or second); yet, all five boys had previously been to camp and were thus aware of "fun things" to do. Ara was the only cabin member to vote on the winning side on all 10 ideas. Omar had the most "wasted" votes, cast for ideas that were not approved by the group, and the most "switch" votes, cast during the second ballot to change from the losing to the winning side. Seven times either Ara or Bjorn said "bad idea" when an activity was suggested; in each case, the activity received no votes, not even from the recommender.

On Day 6 Cabin Two and the brother cabin elected Ara as the tribal chief—a formal recognition of Ara's authority over them as individuals and as a group.

The other Cabin Two boys also revealed characteristic behavior patterns during the first days of camp. The first evening Bjorn wanted to know from SW the exact rules on raids, shaving cream fights, sharing of care packages, etc. The next morning he was the first to talk after the wake-up bell, relating some of the fun things that his cabin had done the previous summer. His leadership recognition in Cabin Two was confirmed by his second place finish in the balloting for tribal chief.

Ernie was the first in the cabin on opening day; he claimed the furthest bunk from the front. Most of his activity during his first several days of camp was done alone—he had places to visit, chipmunks to trap, and trails to investigate. Cabinmates were more than willing to grant Ernie his isolation; Cabin Two became four plus one.

Omar talked incessantly during the first several days, but no one seemed to listen. During free time he followed no one in particular and anyone when he could. By the end of the first week, cabinmates were frequently teasing Omar for talking in his sleep; on several occasions during the camp season Omar woke up with nightmare screams. They also teased him for locking the biffy door when using the facilities; Omar explained that last summer cabinmates did "all sorts of strange things to me when I was in the biffy."

When the group hiked, Omar was in the first or second position 75% of the time. On an intertube trip he floated far ahead of the others: "It gives me a sense of being the leader." One day when he was in the lead, however, and dusk was threatening, he begged SW to take the lead because he was afraid of getting the group lost. Ara and Bjorn were usually in the middle of the group progression, almost never last or next to last—where Ernie was usually located.

The most prominent and intense dyadic relationship in Cabin Two during the first week of camp—and throughout the summer—was between Bjorn and Doug. Friends, school mates, and neighbors for the last several years, the two were keen competitors at camp. Within hours after arrival, the two began their competitive struggle—grabbing chairs out from under each other, fighting with pillows, arguing, flipping towels, and asking where the other had been or was going. Several times their play fights became serious; in most cases Bjorn proved the superior. On Day 11, Bjorn made a policeman's night stick in crafts, "to control Doug." Their dominance encounters constituted over one-third of the total observed in Cabin Two.

There were many times, however, when Doug did not back down from Bjorn—refusing to make bunkbeds, refusing orders, and ridiculing Bjorn's verbal intonations and "goonish" behavior.

The two seldom recognized the other's superior dominance status, but they were frequently physically involved with each other; 65% of all Cabin Two physical assertiveness behavior occurred between Bjorn and Doug. Aside from Bjorn's clear domination over Doug in physical and threat encounters, occurring primarily during clean up and rest hour, the two were essentially equal in status—especially when they argued, ridiculed, and refused each other. Their high level of interactions decreased as camp progressed. By Day 17, Bjorn selected Ara and not Doug as his best cabin friend.

The center of attention quickly shifted from the Bjorn-Doug relationship to Gene on his arrival one week late from hockey camp. The Cabin Two boys remembered Gene as an excellent athlete during the previous summer, so they were looking forward to his arrival. But, Gene brought a style of behavior that spelled chaos. During his first three days at camp he started a small fire on the cabin porch, threw a hockey puck through a cabin wall, and crossed the boy-girl camp border. After one week he was placed on camp probation for physically hurting a boy his age, but of much smaller proportions.

Bjorn and Gene immediately disliked each other. The first breakfast together Gene demanded that Bjorn run for seconds. A surprised and taken aback Bjorn replied, "No!" He shrugged and obeyed. When he returned, Gene immediately demanded more sugar, "since you're up." Bjorn told Gene to "cram it." During clean up later that morning Bjorn ordered Gene to sweep the cabin and chastized him for not flushing the biffy stool. Gene mumbled but followed the directives. Following Bjorn's "victories," others in the cabin stood their ground against Gene's orders and ridicule: Doug threw his socks in Gene's face; Ernie called Gene a dirty name; and Omar refused to help him roll the cabin canvas flaps. By the end of clean up, Gene was subdued.

His first day at camp, Gene was dominant in only eight of his 26 dominance encounters. In the next three days, however, he was dominant in almost 50% of his encounters, dominating Doug, Ernie, and Omar. But against Ara and Bjorn, Gene had little success. His rivalry with Bjorn is reflected in the large proportion of his interactions that were with Bjorn, almost one third. Ara and Bjorn were most successfully dominant over

Gene when giving him directives or when ridiculing him; they seldom engaged him in physical or threat encounters. Levels of interactions with Gene decreased as camp progressed, indicating a resolution of competitive status.

Gene was especially prone to ridicule and physically harass those smaller and weaker than himself, e.g., Omar. During a third week campout the group was finishing the morning pancakes when Gene began his familiar harassment of Omar: name calling and physically nudging. Because his requests to "stop it " were ignored, Omar moved to the other side of the fire where he was greeted with a new challenge: "Afraid of me?" Without warning or precedent, Omar began crying, screaming, and swinging madly and wildly at Gene. He could not allow himself to land the punches—most were aborted hits, never making hard physical contact. For a brief moment Gene was stunned; when he recovered to take revenge, SW intervened. When SW walked with Omar away from the group, Omar's primary concern was that he had violated his conviction of never hitting anyone. After the incident Gene and Omar made a "gentleman's pact" to either ignore or tolerate the other.

For the camp period Omar's most frequent dyadic partner in dominance encounters was Gene. The two were of equal status during verbal arguments and ridicule, but their most frequent mode of interacting was physical assertion, and in these, Gene exerted his dominance over Omar.

Midway through camp, Cabin Two and its brother cabin were involved in a three-way voting deadlock for second half tribal chief among Ara, Bjorn, and Doug. When Bjorn was dropped after the second ballot, Doug won a surprising victory, garnering all the brother cabin votes because, they later told SW, they felt that with Doug they would be more influential in decision making processes.

Doug attempted to be chief—organizing athletic games, assigning swim meet events, etc.—but, despite his legitimatized leadership, few listened or obeyed, especially Ara who maintained cabin leadership, "unofficially." The relationship between the two soured for several days. During the time when Doug was chief, he was never observed to dominate Ara in pair-wise interactions.

As camp progressed to the fourth and fifth weeks, Ara became less actively involved in dominance encounters, but his success percentage rose as he dominated his best friend Bjorn more convincingly than he had before. Counter dominance and recognition behaviors best differentiated the status between them. By the last third of camp Gene was firmly in third place on the dominance hierarchy, capitalizing his upward climb from his first day at camp. Cabinmates recognized this rise. On the Day 17 dominance sociometric his rank order placings ranged from first to last; by Day 28 four placed him second and two fourth, giving him an average slightly greater than Bjorn's average.

During the last third of camp Ernie's success percentage dropped 50% as his encounters with Ara, Bjorn, and Omar decreased in frequency. Ernie seldom interacted with the first two, and was subordinate in 95% of his encounters with them. Doug did not dominate Ernie until the last third of camp, a prominence garnered primarily through verbal directives and ridicules—the same behaviors Ara and Bjorn used to dominate Ernie. Although there was little difference in the dominance status between Ernie and Omar for the camp period, Ernie was dominant during the middle of camp. But by Time Three their level of interacting was less than 1% of the group total.

Thus, by the end of camp relative positions were firmly set, similar to the first week rankings. Fluctuations that occurred were primarily among low ranking group members.

The Data

Almost one third of all dominance behavior observed was verbal ridicule; physical assertiveness was the second most common. Less than 5% of the total was recognition, threat, and displacement behaviors. Of the almost 1200 recorded instances of dominance behavior, 94% was overt in form; as camp progressed overtness increased.

From the first to the middle third of camp there was a slight but nonsignificant increase in the frequency per observation hour of dominance behavoir, but by Time Three the frequency rate had significantly decreased. Daily fluctuations in this frequency rate were rare. The two peak days occurred when Gene arrived at camp on Day 8 and 10 days later when the group went on their two-day campout. Dominance behavior was most likely to occur during athletic games, six times more likely than during mealtimes.

Thirteen of the 15 dyads in Cabin Two were significant in directionality; the Gene-Doug dyad approached significance and the Ernie-Omar dyad was not significant. The former flip-flopped: first Doug, then neither, and then Gene was dominant during the three time periods. Ernie and Omar had few interactions, making any trend in dominance difficult to discern.

The dominance hierarchy increased in stability over time; the number of significant dyads increased from eight to 13 by Time Three. The reversal rate, significant for the camp session, decreased as camp progressed.

The six boys were aware of relative dominance status among themselves. On the three occasions when they ranked each other, their individual listings significantly correlated with each other. These group dominance sociometric rank orders at the beginning, middle, and closing of camp were almost identical to the behaviorally derived dominance hierarchy. In addition, the junior counselor's rankings of the cabin were significantly correlated with the behavioral hierarchy.

The six boys ranked significantly the same regardless of the indice or setting. Ara was first and Omar last or next to last on all indices and settings. Threat and recognition were the best indice predictors of the dominance hierarchy; physical assertiveness and counter dominance, the worse. Athletic games and rest hour-clean up were the best and worst setting predictors, respectively.

High ranking boys in Cabin Six were the leaders of the group, closest to the cabin counselor when sleeping, pubertally advanced for their chronological age, the best athletes, and perceived as the most physically fit; low ranking cabin members were the opposite on these dimensions. Late popularity, physical fitness, and intelligence were highly but nonsignificantly related to the dominance hierarchy.

There was a slight tendency for individuals to interact most with those closest to them on the dominance hierarchy. Three boys were accurate in ranking themselves on dominance; the other three overranked themselves. Best friends were likely to be close in rank and in sleeping position.

Conclusion

Ara's power in Cabin Two was frequently and blatantly demonstrated—and recognized by cabinmates. The theme of the cabin flag was dictated by Ara: C. (Ara's last name) I.A. Ara was president, his name printed in letters twice the size of the other names; below his name was written "Super Agents: Bjorn, SW, Doug." Still further down, in smaller letters Ara wrote, "Agents: Omar, Gene, Ernie." On campouts Omar and Ernie slept next to SW while Ara, Bjorn, Doug and, later, Gene slept side by side.

Ara's position of prominence in the cabin was beneficial to him and to the group. For example, the first day of camp Bjorn did not select his bed until Ara had chosen his. That evening Bjorn started to grab the biggest dish of ice cream but he hesitated, looked at Ara, and then took the second biggest. Several days later Ara knocked over the milk at a lunch meal; Bjorn pointed a condemning finger but, then he apologized, thus preventing potential conflict. The last week of camp Bjorn was conducting a horse 'n goggle when he noticed that Ara was unaware that the extra sandwich was about to be given away. Bjorn did not initiate the procedure until he was sure that Ara was participating.

In addition to directing cabin activities Ara also assumed other prominent roles within the cabin group. When the boys were unable to throw a tire over a tree during Paul Bunyan Day, they turned to Ara, who discovered the method for success. When the group unexpectedly encountered a group of girls on the beach the second week of camp, it was Ara who introduced himself and his cabinmates. He attempted to arrange a rendezvous for that evening between the two groups. For a cabin skit presented before the camp, Ara assumed the primary and only speaking part; Bjorn played a secondary role as the sound effects man.

Many times during the camp session Ara "became" the cabin counselor. When Bjorn and Doug could not agree on the placement of a triple bunk bed, Ara told them where, and the argument was settled. Another time Bjorn gave the peanut butter jar to Ara to open. Gene wanted to order chocolate pudding for the campout but when Ara said, "I don't like chocolate!", the issue was settled. After the cabin group won the first place carnival prize, it was Ara who distributed the candy. Indeed, Ara was occasionally "confused" with SW. Four times Bjorn and once Ernie and Omar referred to SW by Ara's first name. The two names are not phonetically similar.

Perhaps, because of this localization of peer power in one person who maintained an active participation in cabin dominance interactions, there were relatively few problems. The arrival of Gene and his subsequent personality conflicts with Bjorn and Omar and the Bjorn-Doug dyadic confrontations were both settled with minimal disruption of cabin unity. As a result, the group won the all-camp tribal championship by a large margin. This was achieved not solely through athletic games—the team barely won more than it lost—but through Ara's efforts to involve and organize the group in non-athletic camp activities, e.g., cabin inspection.

Cabin Three

Overview

It was an enjoyable summer experience for Cabin Three and their counselor (TS). Cabin authority was exercised almost totally by one boy who maintained that power from the first to the last day of camp. Although there were minor problems during the summer, they were all manageable: one boy's need for attention and affection, a rivalry between two of the campers, and the homesickness of one boy. There were seldom major confrontations between conflicting personalities, only the daily minor hassles caused by irritations and frustrations common among boys living together for five weeks.

The Camp Session

Even though Alex was the authority in Cabin Three, cabinmates were bothered by some of his babyish mannerisms and behavior. Whenever Alex wanted attention he slurred his "r" and "l" sounds, or babbled like a baby. Alex was also prone to crawl on TS's lap or jump on him for a piggy-back ride.

At other times Alex was considerably more "manly." On the amusement park field trip Alex was the only one willing to try all the carnival rides. During cabin play fights he was the only one to actively challenge TS; he kept coming back for more: "Alex doesn't give in to anyone; he's as persistent as hell." On the Day 3 dominance sociometric he was the cabin's choice for most dominant.

Of the 228 dominance encounters occurring during Time One, Alex was a participant in 75% of them as he dominated all cabin members, especially Orville (97%). During the last two-thirds of camp and in seven of the eight indices of dominance behavior he dominated Orville 100% of the time, including all 63 directives and all 34 recognition of status interactions.

By his talk and mannerisms Alex appeared to be the most knowledgeable and experienced boy in Cabin Three; the first year camper Orville was readily responsive to what he said and did. On Day 4 TS noted that Orville was imitating Alex's speech pattern. When Alex told Orville that his nomination for best film stunk, Orville quickly changed his choice. Several times during the first week of camp Orville asked, to no one in particular, "Where's Alex?"

During that first week Orville frequently separated himself from his cabinmates, e.g., sitting apart at meals and moving his sleeping bag away from the rest on campouts. He did not freely participate in cabin play fights, remaining on the periphery of the action. The others laughed at him when he said at the amusement park that he would only ride the ones that "won't make me sick."

Guy was the cabin member most likely to ridicule Orville. On the first day of camp Alex told Guy he was overweight, who replied that Orville, whom he had just met, was fatter. During that first week the two—Guy and Orville—frequently argued as to who was "fattest." Later, their rivalry expanded to include who was the best athlete, who had the best ideas for cabin skits, who ate the best foods, and who had the best hometown. The frequency of dominance interactions between the two was considerably greater than between any other two boys in Cabin Three. During the last two time periods their frequency of interacting was triple the expected rate, over 50% of all dominance encounters occurring in the cabin group. Guy was dominant during all time periods and during cabin discussions. Seventy-two percent of their dominance interactions was either verbal ridicule or argument; Orville was Guy's equal in the latter.

To cabinmates, Guy was lazy and not very intelligent. During cabin conversations and group hikes he lagged behind the others. At the amusement park he sat around, provoking Orville to say, "You never want to do anything. You're too slow and you're always the last one at everything." Guy was an active participant in cabin play fights, until he was hurt; then he withdrew and sulked. The day before the 4th of July

Guy became homesick—staying aloof from the others, not returning their ridicule, and talking about the fun he could be having at home.

After several days Guy "recovered"; from then until the end of camp he became increasingly involved and overt in cabin dominance encounters. Paralleling this increase in participation was a sharp rise in his dominance success percentage, up 18 points by Time Three. By the middle of camp he had replaced Eric as the second most powerful in Cabin Three.

The first few days of camp Eric was friendly and energetic, but also quiet, responsive only when one initiated a conversation with him. Nine days after arrival he was homesick; he requested to be sent home. But, within several days he was again satisfied with camp. TS wrote: "Eric is the hardest person to figure out. He seems to be in his own fantasy world and not really aware of what is going on around him." By the middle of camp Eric was participating in only 10% of the cabin dominance encounters; he fell from the beta to the omega position.

Alex, too, became less involved in cabin interactions during the last weeks of camp. His percentage of participation dropped 22 points during the middle of camp and another 21 points during Time Three. Yet, his success percentage did not decline, rising to over 90% during the last two-thirds of camp. He increased his use of overt strategies of dominating; others, however, became more indirect when dominating him. This was particularly true of his interactions with Guy.

Alex frequently and successfully dominated Guy by verbally directing him, especially during athletic games. Neither was ever observed recognizing the dominance status of the other; however, Alex "won" over 90% of their verbal arguments.

Thus, as camp progressed, Alex solidified his position as the alpha individual in Cabin Three. Guy moved into the number two spot during the middle of camp; the relative dominance status of the other two was never firmly established.

On Day 24 SW, counselor of Cabin Four, and TS switched cabin groups for the day. After the breakfast bell, Alex rushed into the eating lodge and sat beside the guest counselor. Breakfast was relatively quiet except for Alex's recitation to SW of the eating table rules previously established by TS, e.g., finishing firsts before taking seconds, the correct direction to pass food, etc. Eric was especially quiet; not once did he make eye contact with SW.

After breakfast Alex rushed back to the cabin and immediately began sweeping. He instructed the others on their jobs for the day, interrupting SW's "letter writing" to tell him: "Now it's time for the leader to do something. Fill up the water bucket!" Guy appeared tired and passive except when Alex orderd him to sweep and to empty the trash—and when interacting with Orville in a combative spirit.

During lunch the four boys argued as to whether the old table rules were still operative because TS was not there. Alex assured Guy that they were, and he enforced them. Eric attempted to initiate a "sing us a song TS" cheer, but Alex refused to join: "I'm not making a fool of myself." Several moments later, however, it was Alex who started the same yell, with considerably better results (although TS did not sing us a song).

Guy wanted to make bunk beds with Alex during rest hour. Several times Guy, who was 30 pounds heavier, asked Alex for his strength to straighten a bed post. But after Guy was almost finished Alex decided he did not want to sleep in a bunk bed; Guy dismantled what he had completed without complaint. Meanwhile, Orville, who generally was quiet, asked several times for help with his macrame belt; no one responded.

Basketball was the day's athletic game. Alex instructed the others in regard to guarding their opposition and to setting up the offense. Either he or Eric controlled the ball 75% of the time. Guy, near the end of the game, stayed on the offensive end of the court saying that he was too tired to go back and forth. "Besides," he said, "I'm no good on defense and they score every time they get the ball anyway." Cabin Three lost 31-13 as Alex and Eric scored all of the points.

That night at supper Alex determined the order for the horse 'n goggle. The evening cabin discussion was also controlled by Alex, in both content and form—what they would do if they were the camp director.

The Data

Over 75% of the recorded dominance behavior was verbal directives, arguments, and ridicule. No physical assertions or threats were observed. As camp progressed the four boys became significantly more overt in dominating each other; for the camp period two of every three initiated acts were overt.

During the 30 hours of observations, covering 17 days of camp, almost 600 instances of dominance behavior were recorded. There was a slight, but nonsignificant tendency for the per hour rate of observed dominance behavior to decrease as camp progressed. Daily fluctuations in this frequency were slight. There were four peak days of interactions: the first sleep out, the amusement park field trip, and two days in which Guy and Orville argued incessantly. During cabin activities dominance behavior was most likely to occur; discussions and mealtimes had significantly lower frequency rates.

Of the six dyads in Cabin Three, four were significant in directionality. Alex significantly dominated the other three boys and Guy dominated Orville. Eric was placed ahead of Orville because he was dominated by one and not two cabinmates and because he dominated Orville more frequently than vice versa.

Although the reversal rate was significantly low for the camp session, only one of the time periods (One) was significant; the other two approached significance.

The four boys' individual dominance rankings were not significantly interrelated. Alex received three of the four first place votes, and the other three received at least three different positional nominations. The average order of these listings did not correlate highly with the behavioral dominance hierarchy. SW's rankings of the group after he assumed leadership (Day 15 and Day 25) were highly correlated with the behavioral data.

The four boys ranked significantly the same regardless of the setting or indice. Alex ranked first in all settings; rest hour-clean up had the lowest reversal rate. Dominance behavior occurring during cabin activities was the least predictive of the overall order. Verbal ridicule and control were the worst predictors of relative status; recognition, directives, and displacement were the best.

As opposed to low ranking boys, high status individuals in Cabin Three were the youngest and were more likely to interact indirectly rather than overtly. There was no tendency for the boys to interact most with those closest to them on the dominance hierarchy nor to sleep by best friends. Best friends were close in rank.

Conclusion

Alex's authority and power in Cabin Three were frequently "maternal" in form and attitude. During cabin clean up he was in firm control, telling the others how to properly sweep, checking their areas for cleanliness, and enforcing rules on clean up procedures. At lunch on Day 3 he told Orville, "Don't put so much jelly on your bread." Two weeks later when Orville said that he did not like a main dish, Alex told him, "How do you know? You've not even tried it yet. Try it." Alex was consistently monitoring the arguments of Guy and Orville, telling them to "shut up and act your age."

His attitude toward leadership is reflected in his characterization of an ideal leader: "not *too* bossy, tells others where to play, and answers all questions." In Cabin Three he was this kind of a leader. Alex provided an authority that the other boys listened to and obeyed. Even though Eric was a better athlete, Alex told the others—including Eric—where to play, how to play, and for how long. Alex both praised and criticized during athletic games; if criticism, then the others hung their heads. When he was not present during the Day 20 clean up period, little was accomplished and the group received a low inspection score.

Alex's symbol of power was the broom. TS wrote, "The cabin broom has become the symbol of authority. And Alex controls the broom completely." He justified this possession by saying, "I should do most of the sweeping. I'm chief!"

Cabin Four

Overview

It was an unlikely group of four boys who were in Cabin Four: a Midwestern turkey farmer's son; a suburban, one-quarter Native American boy; the son of a business executive; and an urban black. Polite expressions of power during the first week of camp quickly evolved to overt and frequent antagonisms during the remaining four weeks. Play fighting became a way of life in the cabin, first between the low ranking boys and then eventually involving the other two.

Occasionally, play fighting slipped into seriousness. When one became upset or hurt there were quick attempts to patch things, claiming it was only "in fun." A classic struggle for power developed within hours after arrival between a physically aggressive boy and a verbally assertive boy. The battle was settled and all reported having a great time, promising to return the next summer.

The Camp Session

Andy was by nature a physical person; it was a struggle for him to keep his hands to himself as he was always pushing, hitting, pinching, and squeezing cabinmates, SW, and anyone else within his reach. Because of this Andy was immediately disliked by his peers; his bullish behavior was threatening. Soon, whenever he approached, cabinmates cringed, stepped aside, or warned him to leave them alone.

But Andy's "mangling" behavior was rarely intended antagonistically, rather, it was an innocent if misguided attempt to be friendly. But, on occasion, Andy used his physical superiority to threaten cabinmates: "I'm gonna ram this (plunger, broom, etc.) down/up your throat/ass!" No matter how desirable, it was impossible to ignore or avoid Andy. During the first nightly cabin discussion, Andy talked approximately 90% of the time, usually telling stories glorifying his athletic ability, sexual prowess, or personal belongings. Proving his masculinity was a preoccupation. On the first campout he insisted on carrying all cabin equipment in his back pack; he hiked the rougher of two trails, the steeper slope, and the longer route.

It was also apparent that Andy did not particularly like his cabinmates; he made little attempt to get along with them, or even to learn their names. He believed that the camp adminstration would move him to the next oldest unit within a couple of days. This did not materialize.

In contrast to Andy was Otto. When Otto arrived the first day of camp he appeared to be a lost and frightened little boy, hardly one to be in the second oldest age unit. His handshake was weak and his grin was ear-to-ear. Once talking, his high-pitched, shrill voice never stopped—which brought him into immediate confrontation and competition with Andy. It was readily apparent that Otto was well known to returning campers as all called him by a nickname (a small rodent); Otto adopted it when writing his name.

It was Otto's third summer at camp, and he again brought toys from home. This year's special toy was a Goodyear Blimp with a lighted message screen; when playing with it he became totally oblivious to whatever else was occurring in his environment. He also pasted "Fonzie" posters on his trunk and imitated "Fonzie" speech patterns, especially the "hey." Otto was the perfect mascot: fun, energetic, and responsive to all stimuli.

He could be extremely emotional, screaming obscenities, names, and orders, which cabinmates interpreted as aggressiveness during the first week of camp. Andy immediately accepted the challenge. During the first few days of camp the Andy-Otto conflict was bubbling in confrontation. For example, at mealtimes Otto forced Andy to plead before he passed him food; during rest hour he refused to let Andy read his comics or look at his Blimp. In turn, Andy mocked Otto's speech patterns and at mealtimes "accidentally" bumped his arm or leg.

The conflict soon became more overt and intense, especially during athletic games. By verbal directives and physical assertions Andy exerted his power over Otto; Otto's style was to ridicule, counter, refute, and argue. The inevitable crisis came when both were assigned to sweep a building at the end of the first week. Within 10 minutes they were engaged in a vicious broom hitting battle. Because Andy was 55 pounds heavier and eight inches taller, Otto soon returned to the cabin screaming, "I ain't gonna stand that boy bossin' me around; he's got no right and I can't take his shit!" During rest hour later that day Otto flipped an elastic tie band at others in the cabin; all flinched except Andy, who moved closer to him saying, "If you hit me with that I'll wrap it around your neck!"

During Time One the Andy-Otto pair was the most frequently interacting dyad, over twice the expected level. As camp progressed, this level of involvement decreased by 60%, paralleling a 40% increase in Andy's dominance success percentage over Otto. Thus, after many minor fights during the first two weeks the relationship settled into one of mutual toleration, with occasional lapses. For example, during an activity planning meeting Andy changed his vote, thus defeating Otto's plan to visit the craft house. Another day Andy "accidentally" flipped Noxema on Otto, saying, "You were dirty anyway." Otto did most of the avoiding; even though he wanted to assist with the candle shoot-out carnival booth, he volunteered to help with the balloon shaving after discovering that Andy was working on the former.

Rather than interact with Andy, Otto frequently turned to the shy, new camper Delvin. When Delvin entered the cabin on the first day he sauntered to the rear of the cabin to claim his bed. He avoided all eye contact, speaking softly and looking away. His first hour at camp he sat on his bed and watched Otto play, joining only when Otto asked him to help build his Blimp.

When given a choice, Delvin always sat by himself during the first two weeks of camp. At the first cabin meeting he suggested or expressed no ideas or preferences. Because of his small size the others did not recognize his athletic skills—he seemed too small and passive—until the second time period of the first volleyball game. After that he was never again told to "rest" during team games. His buddy Otto told him on Day 7, "Delvin, you need to get out more and meet people."

During the first third of camp Otto was clearly dominant over his friend Delvin. On Day 1 SW asked who would be the table cruiser; Otto pointed at Delvin, even though Delvin had no clue of what to do. When Delvin found loose money in the cabin on Day 4 Otto demanded that he split it with him, which Delvin did without question. Two days later he acccused Delvin of losing his tennis balls, and demanded that he help him look for them, which he did.

But, by the end of the second week Delvin, perhaps because he now felt comfortable in the new environment or because he now too interpreted Otto's agonistic language as only bluff, asserted himself. While Otto was using the biffy one day Delvin hid his surfboard and tennis balls; it soon became a daily all-cabin activity to tease Otto by hiding his prize possessions. On Day 12 Delvin, with the aid of Andy and Gar, threw all of Otto's belongings out of the cabin during rest hour, including his bed and trunk. On Day 15 Otto was upset because his Crazy Machine was missing; he suspected Delvin, who asserted his innocence: "I always thought at first Otto that you'd be a true friend, but now I don't know."

Several days later Gar told SW, "You know, if talking, Otto is tops; if fighting, then Delvin." The data confirmed this observation. Otto dominated Delvin during verbal directive, threat, control, and ridicule behaviors, but Delvin was more dominant in refusing to obey directives, in physically asserting himself, and in displacing Otto. In settings where physical behavior was least possible (discussions and mealtimes) Otto was dominant; during athletic games and activities Delvin ruled the dyad. By the middle of camp their level of interactions had increased 10 percentage points to become the most frequent in Cabin Four. Now Delvin was slightly more dominant; by the last third of camp his success percentage against Otto rose to a highly significant level, primarily through physical assertions.

Otto dropped from the number two to the last place position during the middle third of camp; his success percentage declined by over 40%. Once in that status postion he became more popular with cabinmates. Delvin's pattern was the opposite: as he rose in status his popularity tumbled.

Gar replaced Otto in the runner-up position. It was Gar's fourth summer at camp, and finally he was in the age unit of his dreams—"You always have a blast this year!" The first week of camp Gar knew where to go and what to do, essentially ignoring cabinmates as he visited old places and friends. His longevity at camp should have entitled him to a position of leadership, but Andy's presence thwarted it. Gar wanted leadership, but others were seldom willing to entrust it to him because they felt that he was irresponsible.

Gar was excluded from the cabin play fights because, the others claimed, he did not know how to play fight without becoming overly upset. He usually watched from the periphery, giving a running commentary on the progress of the battle. Gar enjoyed camp because he did not have to be serious, clean, or responsible.

As camp progressed he became more actively involved in dominance encounters. With this increase came a meteoric rise in his dominance success percentage, doubling from Time One to Time Three; this participatory and success increase can be attributed to his interactions with Otto. Although the two were infrequent interactors during Time One, by Time Two they had doubled their participatory level, and by the last third of camp no dyad was interacting more frequently. Now, Gar was clearly more dominant, achieved primarily through counter dominance, threat, and physical assertive behaviors.

Gar was the only member who, on occasion, challenged Andy. Even though the two rarely fought, one day Andy overstepped when he dumped cold water on Gar to "wake him up" at the close of rest hour. Gar was furious and despite Andy's warning, threw water on him. Andy wrestled him to the floor as the latter yelled, "I give! I give!" Gar was more successful later in camp and when using verbal indices of dominance: demanding an end to Andy's towel flipping on Day 11; chastizing him for missing the stool when he peed on Day 21; and yelling at him for sticking his peanut butter coated knife in the jelly jar on Day 25. However, over the camp period, Gar frequently recognized Andy's superior dominance status. By the last week of camp, Gar selected not his first week friend Delvin, but Andy as his best friend, a reciprocal selection.

The Gar-Delvin friendship emerged when they found a common interest, horseshoes. During the course of camp their level of dominance encounters was the lowest in the cabin. Gar was only slightly dominant over Delvin, primarily during physical assertive and verbal control behaviors and during camp discussions. Delvin was the dominant pair member during mealtimes and when counter dominating.

Delvin's friendship with Gar was the beginning of his "coming out." During a cabin discussion on Day 14 he admitted to the group, "When I talk I'm chicken to speak out so I shut up." It was during one of his many mid-camp play fights with Otto that cabinmates discovered his wrestling ability. Several times he headlocked Otto, and once Andy. Yet, Delvin retreated from Andy despite his superiority in fighting ability. Delvin's increased status culminated in his unexpected election as the second half tribal chief. Both his involvement in and his success at dominance encounters increased 20 percentage points by the last third of camp.

The cabin "scapegoat" thus switched from Delvin to Otto during the course of camp. When hiking, the cabin progression was usually Andy in front, followed by Gar, Delvin, and Otto. More than anyone else, Delvin yelled at Otto for lagging behind. Otto was usually last because he could not carry his equipment, made heavier by "unneeded" items (pillow, radio, toys). In order to sleep at night Otto had to have these items, and to habitually bang his head against a pillow or to rock his legs or body back and forth. The others ignored this habit, but Delvin criticized it ("You could really stop it if you really wanted to."), despite Otto's apologies—he had had the habit since he was a baby.

All enjoyed teasing Otto about his fear of the night. On campouts, they howled like wolves or screamed that they were being eaten alive by spiders and rats. This teasing was usually sufficient to elicit crying, necessitating SW's intervention. One evening Otto woke SW to tell him that there were strange animals outside trying to come into the cabin. Rational assurances did little to ease his fears. Only when SW moved his bed closer to Otto did he fall asleep. Otto's other irrational fear was water. During the swim test he panicked, screaming, "Mommy! Mommy!" The water was not over his head and a life guard pole was inches from him. Delvin mockingly reminded Otto of this incident several times during camp.

By the last week of camp Andy was clearly the most dominant boy in Cabin Four. The others had adjusted to his physical behavior and to his boasting. But Andy was spending less time with the group; his participation in cabin dominance interactions dropped by one-third during the last half of camp. He loved going to the beach around sunset; if left alone he would sit there for hours, returning to the group reflective and calm. When with the group he was an active participant in cabin play fights—which communicated to the other boys that his physical behavior was not usually intended for harm's sake.

The Data

Verbal ridicule was the most common category of dominance behavior observed in the cabin and physical assertion was a close second. Threat, displacement, and recognition behaviors comprised only 11% of the total.

Of the 1600 recorded instances of dominance behavior, almost 90% was categorized as overt. The proportion of overt to indirect behavior significantly increased from Time One to Time Three.

The per hour frequency rate, which was the highest of any observed cabin group, increased dramatically as camp progressed. There were several days when the frequency rate skyrocketed, all occurring after the first third of camp. On all five occasions the Cabin Four boys were teasing Otto: hogtieing, seed spitting, pillow fighting, throwing possessions, etc. These play fights occurred during rest hour or clean up. Bedtimes and mealtimes were peaceful behavior settings.

Four of the six dyadic relationships were significant in directionality after five weeks of camp. Andy was the top ranked individual throughout camp, but the other three boys shifted positions—Otto falling from the number two to the fourth position during the middle of camp with the two boys formerly under him in rank each moving up one notch.

It is only when behavior occurring during the last third of camp is considered, does the percentage of transgressions against the hierarchy become significantly less than behavior congruent with a hierarchical arrangement of group members. During this time five of the dyads were significant in directionality. For the entire five weeks of camp the reversal rate was signficantly low.

The boys' individual listings of relative dominance status were not significantly interrelated on Day 3, but by the end of camp there was general agreement as to the dominance hierarchy. Furthermore, this dominance sociometric ordering was significantly correlated with the behavioral dominance hierarchy. Nongroup adults ranked the cabin on Day 4, 16, and 19; all were significantly similar to the behavioral hierarchy of Time One, Two, and Three, respectively.

The four boys ranked significantly the same regardless of the indice of dominance behavior used to rank order them or the behavior setting in which they were observed. Physical assertion best predicted the overall dominance hierarchy; counter dominance and verbal control were the worse predictors. Behavior occurring during athletic games was predictive of dominance status; mealtime behavior was not.

The boys' rankings on physical size, socioeconomic status, hiking position, and usage of indirect indices of dominance behavior were predictive of relative dominance status. High ranking boys also tended to be more physically attractive and pubertally advanced, and to be the leaders of the group and to sleep furthest from the counselor. Best friends were both close in rank and in bed position. There was no relationship between dominance rank and whom one interacted with most frequently.

Conclusions

Perhaps because of his status position Andy usually received what he wanted. On Day 1 he let it be known that he was going to sit beside SW during meals, and he maintained that position throughout camp. On Day 10 Delvin had a choice of passing the cake, and, hence, decide who would grab the second largest piece, to Andy or to his best friend Otto. He passed it to Andy. When Gar suggested on Day 16 that perhaps the defense and the offense could switch for one day, Andy ended the egalitarian effort by retorting, "Hell, no one is going to stick me on defense!" When Andy was in the top bunk, Gar frequently complained that his feet were hanging over the side of the bed in his face. Andy's usual response was "Tough! Move your face." After they switched positions at mid-camp, Gar quickly moved his feet when Andy complained that they were in his face.

The Cabin Four boys were physically afraid of Andy, especially Delvin. Even though Delvin was the superior towel flipper, Andy backed him into a corner, flipping his towel more frequently and harder. On a Day 24 campout Andy suggested "King of the Hill"; Delvin hollered, "Oh, no!" as he ran away. Later Delvin remembered that he "owed" Andy a hit; he approached, but backed away when Andy stood and dared him.

The others only got "even" when Andy could not defend himself. For example, one evening when Andy was late for supper the others insinuated, with an obvious attempt to increase his chances of getting in trouble, that he was at girls' camp, "doing it to them." On the sociometrics the group described Andy in negative terms; although Delvin always said that Andy was the leader of the group, he rated him a "D+" on the leadership sociometric.

Andy's presence was benefical to the group. Even though Delvin was obviously the better athlete and knew more about the athletic game being played, only Andy was able to tell the others where and how to play the position, and who yelled instructions that organized the group into a coherent whole. Even after Delvin became the tribal chief during the last half of camp, Andy was still the directing and organizing force.

When the group was away from the cabin, Andy served as the regulator of expected behavior. On a campout he instructed the others on various camping skills, cooking the supper meal when he saw that Gar did not know what to do. Andy organized turn-taking in stirring the supper stew, an unenviable job because of the heat and smoke. No one suggested that he should also stir.

Andy automatically assumed the role of cabin rule enforcer and leadership representative. The first day of camp he told Otto to take off his baseball cap in the eating lodge. After SW told everyone that they had to finish whatever food they placed on their plates, Andy told Gar to drink his milk and Otto to drink his juice. Whenever there was extra desirable food, Andy regulated the random process of distribution, the horse 'n goggle. During cabin clean up on Day 26, he ordered the others to stop playing around because inspection was worth double that day— and he told SW to sweep the trail path, and to do a good job! When the cabin needed a representative before the entire camp, Andy volunteered, even though it was rightly Delvin's job as chief, e.g., selecting the cabin's lottery number for the special 4th of July activity.

The flavor of the dominance relations in Cabin Four can best be illustrated, and summarized, by reference to the cabin flag making exercise.

Andy immediatly grabbed the flag cloth and penciled a design; he turned to Gar for advice, but none was given. Otto shouted several moments later, "I didn't say ya could do it!" Ignoring this interference, Andy wrote the tribal name at the top of the flag. Meanwhile, Delvin and Otto were throwing sticks at each other with Gar watching and giggling. SW suggested that all should participate by drawing a design proposal on paper and the winning one, as determined by group vote, would be drawn on the flag. Otto's design was unintelligible and neither Delvin's sunset nor Gar's bicentennial flag aroused enthusiasm. Andy, who had not participated in the "contest," now drew a bicentennial sunset; it was readily accepted by the others. Without consultation, Andy drew his design as Gar and Delvin watched. Gar suggested an alteration but Andy told him "stupid idea," and continued drawing. Otto, who had been playing in the fireplace, came over and screamed, "I didn't tell ya to draw that you bastard Andy!" Andy's reply was almost predictable, "Tough shit boy!" Gar said that everyone should color; Andy agreed: "Gar, you color the water. Otto, you do the sun." Otto asked how and Andy demonstrated. Then, Andy decided "mountains would be nice" and he told Gar to add them. But, when Gar said that he did not know how, Andy grabbed the crayon and drew them. When the flag was near completion Andy printed names on the flag. Delvin objected that everyone should print his own name so as to add a sense of involvement. Andy told each of them the color and size of print. Andy, whose name was already on top, told SW, "I'm writing your name on the bottom." Everyone left, leaving the mess and SW.

5
Life in the Female Cabin Groups

Cabin Five

Overview

The five girls in Cabin Five experienced few major problems during their five weeks together. Cabin authority and power were primarily invested in one girl who indirectly asserted herself during the first week of camp, and then effectively withdrew from active participation in group power struggles until the last days of camp when her authority was challenged. In the interim, more assertive and overt dominance acts pervaded cabin life, especially directed against a vulnerable, submissive girl. Power status was recognized and stabilized at the poles, top and bottom, and three girls fluctuated within the middle ranks of dominance status. The cabin counselor, CH, wrote after the camp session: "While there were problems every day, we managed to survive the five weeks; others were not so lucky."

The Camp Session

Meeting Amy on Day 1, CH was immediately struck by her aura of self-confidence and calm: "She does not appear in the least to be disturbed by the tumultuous first day chaos." Amy greeted old friends with shrieks and hugs, whispering and giggling with each of them. When with the cabin, an infrequent occurrence during the first few days, Amy was more subdued, but still social; she talked to everyone and expected an answer, which she inevitably received. Reminding the others of her previous camp experience, Amy was the source of knowledge and gossip: "She knows the ropes and no one gives her trouble.", CH wrote in her observation notebook. When cabinmates asked questions "in general," Amy answered, frequently interrupting CH. During cabin meetings nine out of 10 times Amy dictated both the suggested activities and their acceptance. Most mornings Amy assumed the critical director's role for cabin clean up; if someone was tardy in her assigned task, then Amy did it for her. Thus, other Cabin Five girls felt guilty because they now owed her a favor. At the end of the first week Gilda told CH, "I try to be perfect like her (Amy), but I just can't do everything right like she does, and I'm tired of feeling bad about it."

In contrast to Amy was Betty, also a returning camper, who was not enthusiastic in greeting last summer's friends. With her new cabinmates she was cool, aloof, and tolerant. She associated with a neighboring cabin group or walked alone, slumped forward with arms folded across her chest. When with Cabin Five, Betty relentlessly ridiculed the other girls, especially Olivia. Gilda called Betty, "Little Miss Mature"; Gilda continually sought her as an audience for her steady stream of jokes and antics. Betty was sometimes attentive, sometimes polite, and, frequently, not interested.

Amy and Betty were neither good friends nor mutual associates. They seldom sat together, essentially ignoring each other; they averaged less than two dominance interactions per day from Day 4 to Day 26. During the first and last three days of camp Amy dominated Betty in almost 90% of their interactions, primarily through verbal arguments and physical assertiveness. Betty recognized the superior dominance status of Amy almost three times more frequently than Amy did hers. On Day 6 Amy and Betty could not decide who should take the bigger of the two doughnuts that remained. Amy eventually ordered, "Take one, will you!" Betty shrugged and took the *smaller.*

The behavior of Gilda and Donna during the first week of camp spanned quite variant styles of interacting. Gilda craved attention; she threw water balloons and knocked over things during mealtimes while grabbing, too impatient with the slower and more polite methods of table graces. On the other hand, Donna, as a newcomer to camp, was terribly shy the first few days of camp, rarely stretching beyond her primary base of support, the cabin. She was quiet, almost nonexistent. Participating in few dominance encounters, Donna was rarely the dominant member in pair-wise interactions with cabinmates.

Olivia was a special case. From the first moments of camp she seemed to invite and even encourage taunting and ridicule. To cabinmates Olivia was an embarrassment, someone uncool. CH was not sure what it was about Olivia that elicited such universal reaction—perhaps her many questions, her hoarding of her belongings, her childish and brattish manner of interacting with peers, and her persistent and nagging ever-presence. She followed the others around like a shadow; some said she was a leech. When something was said in her presence she assumed—with good reason—that it was a vicious slam against her. Despite her boisterous appearance and mannerisms, she spoke so softly that it was often difficult to comprehend what she was saying.

Betty was Olivia's most persistent and cruel tormentor, dominating her in all settings, utilizing most indices, during the entirety of camp. Olivia initiated more recognition behavior in the presence of Betty than she did to the other three girls combined. Amy, Gilda, and Donna also dominated Olivia during all three time periods and most behavior settings. Donna was the only Cabin Five girl who did not frequently dominate Olivia, the girl who Olivia sat beside most frequently.

During the third week of camp a friendship between Amy and Donna developed; they frequently sat beside each other and whispered. For the first time Amy was dominant over Donna. And, too, CH noted that Donna began to "come out" more. During the last two weeks of camp Donna initiated one-half of her directive, ridicule, and physical assertive behaviors, and received slightly over 50% of cabinmates' recognition of status behaviors. Her success rate increased by 60% and she was dominated only by Amy.

In particular, Donna's relationship with Betty was altered. Previously, Betty dominated her but during the last two weeks of camp Donna maneuvered around or through Betty's taunting, often ordering her to stop. Now they were of equal status. Donna used indirect strategies to dominate Betty; Betty was more overt toward Donna than she was to any other Cabin Five girl. This overtness level, however, dropped 80% during the time when the two were of equal status.

CH felt that Donna rose in status as a direct consequence of her association with Amy: Others responded to her as an extension of Amy's power and authority. Perhaps Donna's assertion of power reflected her growing familiarity with the new camp surroundings and with her experience in living with four other girls. The friendship could, thus, be interpreted as an attempt by Amy to thwart a potential threat to her status, thus preserving and solidifying her own position through a coalition with Donna.

This latter interpretation fits Amy's pattern of relating: She first established domination over a girl, withdrew from such encounters, and renewed it again only if the relationship required reinforcing. Amy dominated Gilda during the first third of camp, and then seldom interacted with her during the rest of camp. During the last three days of camp Amy renewed dominance interactions with Betty, matching in three days the number of encounters that had occurred between the pair during the preceding two weeks.

Throughout camp Betty maintained her cabin respect, becoming less mysterious after the first two weeks when she began to laugh, smile, and interact in a friendly fashion with the other Cabin Five girls. She also increased by 50% her participation in cabin dominance encounters, paralleling Amy's "disinvolvement." But, during the last few days of camp Betty became "frustratingly and frighteningly" powerful over the other girls: taunting Olivia, horseplaying with Gilda, and shunning Amy and Donna. CH recorded the following impression:

For some time Betty appeared to have much potential power, especially a strange way of mystifying us all, and toward the last days her sultriness, taunting, and cattiness really came out. She especially took pleasure in someone else's misfortunes—often laughing at anyone who lost something, broke something, spilt something, or forgot something.

It was during these "last days" when Amy changed from her previous pattern of ignoring Betty to actively dominating her. Amy, thus, moved from the beta position during the middle of camp to most dominant, her Time One position.

Amy and Betty, however, combined forces during a last week "emergency." CH's glasses were lost in the lake and she was left "blind"; Amy and Betty immediately took charge, working together to organize duties to be assumed by other girls for the beach night supper. They were the list makers, the directors who advised Gilda and Donna on constructing and starting the camp fire and in cooking, and who told Olivia where the best firewood could be found.

During this last week of camp Gilda became increasingly aggressive in her talk, horseplay, and jokes. But, she also spent increasing amounts of time by herself, frequently leaving the cabin group for extended periods of time. Her involvement in cabin dominance encounters declined 10 percentage points during the last third of camp, and her dominance success percentage dropped 30 points as she only dominated Olivia. Previously, she was equal in rank with Betty. During a nine day period at the end of the second time period Betty clearly dominated Gilda through ridicule and counter dominance. The level of dominance interactions between the two was the highest in the cabin, doubling in frequency from the first to last time periods.

As Gilda withdrew, so too did Olivia, into her own world. Within the cabin group Olivia had no niche. When she led no one followed; when she joked no one laughed; and when she ordered no one obeyed. Starved for attention, when Betty asked to borrow a tee shirt for the banquet, Olivia was so thrilled by this recognition that she proceeded to become Betty's servant, holding a small mirror while Betty preened herself. Camp had taught Olivia not to be so obnoxious and blatant; toward Betty's vicious tongue she had developed a "turning the other cheek" approach. To survive the five weeks Olivia had to change her behavior; she did the minimum.

The last few days of camp were especially difficult for Cabin Five. CH wrote: "I feel like these last three days have been a CONSTANT battle to keep the five girls from splittering...almost as though a lid had been removed from above these five kids and all their storm poured out in one great three day blast." The frequency of interactions during the last four days was 75% higher than the overall five week frequency average.

Time together as a cabin group apparently had some effect: Amy mellowed in her domination; Betty joined the group in spirit; Gilda became less rowdy and more lonely; Donna developed a friendship with Amy; and Olivia learned how not to get on everyone's nerves.

The Data

Directive, ridicule, and recognition behaviors accounted for nearly 75% of the total number of dominance interactions recorded; 57% were overt. But, during the course of the camp session the proportion of indirect behaviors significantly increased, to the point that indirect expressions of dominance behavior outnumbered the direct during the last third of camp.

The per hour frequency of dominance interactions did not significantly change during the camp period; during the middle of camp the frequency was highest. Daily fluctuations in the per hour frequency rate was common; peaks corresponded to important events occurring during camp. For example, the highest daily average, almost three times the overall average, was on Day 27, the all-camp banquet. Other peaks occurred when Amy received a letter detailing her parents' divorce and when CH's Chicago boyfriend visited her. Dominance behavior was most likely to occur during cabin activities and clean-up; mealtimes were the most peaceful settings.

All 10 dyads in Cabin Five were significant in directionality. Amy dominated the other four girls; Betty, all but Amy; Gilda, Donna and Olivia; and Donna, Olivia. The percentage of interactions that transgressed this hierarchical arrangement was relatively small (23%) and statistically less than hierarchical congruent behavior.

But a detailed temporal analysis of the data reveals fluctuations in the hierarchy. During Time One Betty and Gilda were of equal status, thus creating a two-way tie for second place. Betty then rose to the top position, exchanging postions with Amy during the middle of camp, creating another two-way tie for second place (with Gilda). Amy regained alpha status during the last third of camp; Donna rose from fourth to a two-way tie with Betty for second place; Gilda fell to fourth; and Olivia remained her usual fifth.

The agreement among these three time rankings barely reached significance. Even though the reversal rate was significantly low in all three time periods, clearly the hierarchy was prone to alterations.

The behavioral rank ordering was not recognized by the five girls on the Day 3 sociometric. Neither did their individual listings significantly correlate with each other. The junior counselor's assessment of the cabin's dominace hierarchy agreed with neither the behavioral nor the sociometric orderings.

The five girls ranked significantly the same regardless of the indice or behavior setting. There was an inverse relationship between good prediction and frequency rate, i.e., the more frequently a particular indice of behavior (directives) was observed or the more frequently dominance behavior occurred in a particular behavior setting (clean up) then the more likely was that indice or behavior setting to be a good predictor of the Cabin Five dominance hierarchy (to have a low reversal rate).

Advanced age and high intelligence significantly correlated with dominance in Cabin Five. High ranking girls also tended to be more physically mature and of lower SES standing than were low ranking members, who had the most accurate assessment of the dominance hierarchy. There was no consistent tendency for the girls to have the most interactions with those closest to them in the hierarchy or for dominance status and frequency of engagement in dominance behavior to be related.

Conclusion

It was difficult for CH to assess who was most dominant in Cabin Five:

I really am unsure as to who is calling the shots. Each day I feel as though a new set of rules is being shaped, or a new face is up front. Here it is each for herself. These kids confuse me; I don't think any one of them is 'most' dominant.

CH portrayed Amy as a maternal/martyr type; Betty was more of an antagonistic, up-front girl.

Amy's style was to give directives; Betty's was to ridicule and to counter cabinmates. Amy's demands were seldom argued as she got her way most of the time, especially when interactions occurred within the cabin. The other girls described her as "self-assured, experienced, knowledgeable, mellow, mature, and quiet." As Amy withdrew from active participation in cabin dominance encounters, Betty was quick to fill the void, becoming more involved as camp progressed. When the group was away from the cabin, then Betty was the most prominent girl, exerting power in an overt and antagonistic manner. Cabinmates described her as "insecure, aloof, fake, manipulative, and strong."

Within the cabin Amy controlled the nature of power relations. For example, her coalition with Donna brought the latter to a new position of prominence during the last week of camp. But, when she became an absentee during the middle of camp, Betty, the mood setter, assumed charge.

Cabin Six

Overview

Cabin Six had two major difficulties: one girl reknowned for the frequent and assertive manner in which she expressed her power and another girl unable to defend herself against verbal and physical assaults. As the summer progressed, living together became a more pleasant experience for the five girls, primarily because a first year camper gradually exerted the necessary control over the assertive girl in a fashion conducive to effective and cooperative authority and leadership. The vulnerable girl learned during the five weeks how to defend herself and how to cope with living in a group; in turn, cabinmates became more tolerant of her.

The Camp Session

During the first week of camp Becky was the "match under the firecracker," and her independence and charisma often brought near riot conditions within the cabin. For example, one evening she entered the cabin popping gum, squirting a water gun, and initiating with her friend from last year's group, Gloria, a pillow and water fight. From the first morning Becky behaved as if she were the ultimate source of power and authority within the cabin: "We don't have to get up now and clean up because there's no inspection on the first day." During cabin clean up she refused to do jobs requested by CW, and then she proceeded to tell the others how to do their jobs.

At the beginning of camp Becky's authority was unquestioned. One morning CW suggested to the cabin that they plan a vesper service for the entire camp. After a moment of silence Becky groaned and the cabin in unison shouted "No!" During the first three days of camp her dominance success rate was the highest in the cabin; Becky was clearly the most dominant girl in Cabin Six.

Becky's most responsive audience was Dottie who gave more recognition behaviors to Becky than any Cabin Six member gave to another. More than anything else, Dottie wanted to avoid being a "nobody." By responding to the antics of Becky and Gloria she received attention and some measure of acceptance. Dottie laughed at any joke and followed any act. One day she lied to protect Becky; later that day she cried, confessing to CW that she had compromised her moral principles. To CW Dottie had little backbone, no will power or sense of self:

Dottie continues to be the follower of whoever is in command at the moment. She is immature, insecure, and wants be remain in everyone's favor regardless of the cost. She is so sensitive to everything around her that it is hard to believe she is insensitive to the way others treat her.

Whenever Dottie received a care package from home she immediately shared its contents—candies and cookies.

Dottie displayed many of the stereotypic gestures and ritualistic behaviors of subordinates: giving food away, moving from the path of higher status girls, always smiling, offering favors, and watching others to monitor their reactions. She gave 50% of all recognition behaviors observed in Cabin Six. She dominated only Opal and this percentage decreased 25 points during Time Three when Opal countered Dottie's constant directives and ridicules with verbal arguments.

Opal was a complainer and a negativist. Beginning with the first day of camp, Opal was a prime recipient of teasing and taunting, occasionally cruel in nature. For example, Gloria asked Becky, in the presence of Opal, what she thought of those who "look retarded with heads larger than their bodies—you know, little stubby bodies."

When Opal did not get her way she pouted and whined, withdrawing to the periphery of the group. She was also a clinger, physically attaching herself to any leader who blessed her with attention. On the first cabin campout Opal slept closest to CW; the other four girls slept on the other side of the camp fire. One of CW's leader friends wrote that Opal looked and acted like a sad, Peanuts-type character: "She's a kind of a loser, but she holds on nicely."

Only Gloria during the first week challenged Becky's authority, usually in a friendly, teasing manner. Even though Gloria frequently joined Becky in her many antics, Becky initiated, went further, and did not stop. After the first week of camp CW wrote, "Gloria is the quiet one with the unrealized leadership potential."

In direct contrast to Dottie's and Opal's attempts to become a part of the Becky-Gloria circle was Ann's reactions during the first week of camp. Unlike other first year campers, Ann did not simply follow her more experienced peers to and from camp activities; rather, she lagged behind, exploring the camp grounds on her own. By the end of the first week she emerged from the self-imposed protective shell. Although still marginal to the group, Ann was included by Becky and Gloria in their pillow fights; she frequently asked them for advice and information.

Ann did not so readily submit to Becky's commands as did the others. On Day 2 Becky jokingly told Ann to peel an orange for her because she was busy doing her nails. Ann hesitatingly agreed, but pretended to spit on the orange, thus literally obeying but still winning half the battle. By the second week Ann no longer waited for Becky to wake up before beginning her morning cleanup duties. In the evenings she frequently asked Becky to be quiet so that she could sleep. Soon, Ann defended herself in pillow fights, if not physically then verbally by threatening Becky and Gloria. By the end of the third week it became apparent that Ann was waging a subtle, and yet most effective, anti-Becky campaign within the cabin. In front of Becky she said she had no complaints, but behind her back she told the other girls that Becky was the source of cabin dissension. When Becky lied to CW about doing her cleanup job one day, Ann "finked" on her.

The level of interactions between Ann and Becky was the second highest in the cabin. Although Becky was dominant over Ann after the first three days of camp, from Day 4 through Day 23 the two were equal in their dyadic interactions.

Once Ann increasingly challenged Becky's power, the other Cabin Six girls complained, first to CW and then in the presence of the total group, about Becky's insensitivity to their feelings and her disruptive, chaotic behavior. A week earlier the girls willingly made excuses for Becky. On Day 7 CW explained to Becky the necessity of attending all-camp events; two hours later she skipped the requried church service. When CW confronted Becky, the other girls defended her; "She didn't hear the bell!" They said that they did not mind waiting for Becky when she woke up late, did not complete her cleanup tasks on time, and was tardy for meals and activities. But, as camp progressed the girls grew to like Becky less and less: On the Day 28 sociometric, Opal kept her as her least best friend; Dottie dropped her one notch; and Ann and Gloria who had earlier placed Becky as their best friend, dropped her to third and second, respectively.

The strain between Gloria and Becky became most explicit by the last third of camp. Gloria blocked Becky's bed rearrangement plan because she did not want to forfeit her ideal position. Their peak conflict came during the fourth week when Gloria planned to visit another cabin for several days—an allowable event for one cabin member during a summer. When Becky heard of this she decided to do likewise, going to the camp director before Gloria did. Gloria did not complain of this usurpation until she discovered that Becky had known of her plans. After several meetings with the camp director concerning the "misunderstanding," Gloria vowed that Becky would not get away with her "dirty tricks."

As camp progressed Gloria participated less frequently in Becky's games, preferring instead to be alone or with Ann. Their level of interactions, the most frequent of any dyad in the cabin, dropped 75% during the last third of camp. Excluding the first three days of camp, Becky did not establish a consistent domination pattern over Gloria. Becky was more dominant when employing physical assertive behaviors and Gloria dominated Becky by ignoring and refusing requests.

The strained relationship between Ann and Becky became overt during the last week of camp. After Becky and Gloria selected a spot for the last beach night supper, Ann said that she would rather eat on the sand dunes. After faces and grumblings Becky, and then the rest of the girls, followed Ann's lead. The next morning Ann condemned Becky for her constant put-downs of Opal; Becky stomped out of the cabin. The last night of camp Ann did not want to sleep out and, after arguing with Becky, she suggested a compromise: They would eat on the beach but come in to sleep. Becky begrudingly accepted this solution to the impasse.

By the last week of camp Ann was the best liked girl in Cabin Six, everyone's, except Becky's, best friend. Earlier, during the first week of camp, she was the third best liked in the cabin. In particular, Gloria described Ann in glowing terms: the cabin leader, dominant, friendly, pretty, smart, and popular. During the last 10 days of camp Ann's involvement in cabin dominance encounters rose dramatically (66%) as she, for the first time, dominated both Becky and Gloria. This domination was achieved primarily through indirect forms of ridicule (gossip), directives (suggesting behavior), and verbal control (corrections) and the overt use of physical play fighting. Ann's control over Dottie and Opal was primarily maintained through verbal directives during clean up and mealtimes. The interactions betweeen Ann and Dottie increased during this time—equaling the combined total of the first two-thirds of camp—primarily the result of Dottie recognizing Ann's new position of authority in the cabin. Ann's success percentage rose steadily through camp, from 53% to 69% to 89% during the three time periods.

This rise in Ann's status paralleled Becky's decline, a drop of 24 points during the last 10 days of camp. Also occurring during this last week was an alteration in Dottie's behavior. Her involvement in cabin dominance interactions spiraled upward as camp progressed, almost doubling from the first to the last third of camp. By Time Three she had superseded Becky as the cabin's most actively involved in dominance encounters. Dottie maintained a good relationship with Opal through most of camp—consistent with her desire to keep friendly relations with everyone—but by the end of camp she became impatient with and vindictive toward Opal. This was in direct contrast to the other girls' reactions toward Opal. Over time they became more tolerant of her, not necessarily friendly and yet no longer hostile.

During the last two weeks of camp Opal became considerably more friendly, and at times more assertive. More involved and overt in dominance interactions, Opal doubled her Time One success percentage, primarily through arguing with Dottie during cabin discussions. She still frequently imitated those of high status. For example, in preparing for the all-camp banquet she combed her hair exactly as Ann did.

The Data

Three categories of behavior—ridicule, directive, and recognition—together represented over 75% of the dominance observed in Cabin Six. Threats and displacements were rare events. From the first to the third time periods the recorded dominance behavior became progressively more indirect; overall, more behavior was indirect (53%) than direct.

The frequency rate of dominance behavior rose during the last 10 days of camp when Ann exerted her dominance over Becky and Gloria. There were relatively few dramatic fluctuations in the daily frequency rate, peaking the day of and the day after the all-camp banquet. Besides being the most unstable setting (a high reversal rate) cabin discussions were also a time when the frequency rate was highest. Mealtimes and clean up were more peaceful.

Overall, eight of the 10 dyads were statistically significant in directionality. Only two girls—Dottie and Opal—were firmly positioned early in camp, not varying by time, setting, or indice. At the onset of camp Becky was the alpha individual, dominating both Ann and Gloria after three days of camp. There was no status difference between Ann and Gloria. The three soon became equal in rank, remaining so until the last week of camp when Ann's dominance over both Becky and Gloria became statistically significant. Becky's dominance over Gloria approached signficance for the camp session.

Overall, the reversal rate (28%) was significantly lower than hierarchical harmonious behavior. This percentage decreased steadily over time, indicating an increasing recognition of status differential among the five girls.

The five girls ranked significantly the same regardless of indice or behavior setting. Verbal ridicule and directive behaviors and clean up activity settings had the lowest reversal rates, i.e., the best predictors of the overall dominance hierarchy.

When the Cabin Six girls ranked each other on relative dominance, their individual listings were significantly intercorrelated on both Day 3 and Day 28. Their group order had Becky placed in the first position, Gloria in second, Ann in third, Dottie in fourth, and Opal in fifth. Nongroup observers rank ordered the girls in the same relative positions.

The most dominant girls in Cabin Six were athletic and pubertally advanced, but they were not the oldest nor the largest in the cabin. There was a tendency for the high ranking individuals to be popular and to be more actively involved in cabin dominance encounters than low ranking girls. Cabin Six girls usually interacted most with those closest to them in hierarchical rank. All but Ann and Opal overranked themselves on the dominance sociometric. Best friends were close in rank on Day 4; this was not true by the end of camp.

Conclusions

When CW asked the girls at the close of camp who was the cabin mood setter, Becky replied: "I hope you don't think I'm being conceited or anything, but I think I am!" No one disagreed. Throughout camp Becky was known as a "problem." A fellow leader told CW after the first week of camp that Becky was skipping athletic games; another told her the next week that Becky was smoking in the woods.

Of the five girls Becky was the most overt and involved in dominance interactions. It was not until the last week of camp when Ann rose to prominence that Becky was involved in less than two of every three dominance encounters occurring in Cabin Six. Despite Opal's low status and threat potential, Becky dominated her frequently and overtly throughout camp, primarily through a relentless barrage of directives, taunts, and teases. Becky was the unanimous choice for cabin bully.

In direct contrast was Ann's style of authority; subtle and manipulative, she became the cabin's "mother." She instructed the others on cleanup jobs, corrected Opal's table manners ("Dottie, pass Opal a napkin so she can wipe the jelly off her face."), and woke up the group in the morning. Ann worked out a suitable bed arrangement plan, a compromise between the desires of Becky and Gloria.

Ann became powerful in the cabin by first blocking Becky's dominance initiations through refusing and shunning and then through ignoring her during the next three weeks. By the fifth week of camp Ann effectively controlled Becky through physical assertion, ridicule, and directive behaviors. CW wrote during the last week: "Ann has apparently moved up the past couple of days. She enjoys Becky and lets her do her thing, but is not afraid to step in and put her foot down when she feels it is necessary, or to do her thing when it runs counter to Becky's."

To CW, junior counselors, and fellow leaders, the two different styles of "leadership" within Cabin Six were striking. Becky did what she wanted, attracting followers by her personal magnetism and charisma. Ann seemed more aware of her power and used it to manipulate and control others. The newness of the camp setting may have prevented her from a quicker rise to power in the cabin.

Cabin Seven

Overview

The locus of power in Cabin Seven frequently shifted among the five girls: during camp one girl fell three places on the dominance hierarchy, two occupied the top spot at different times, and all were involved in three-way ties for various status positions. There were many compatible moments when the five girls worked together, especially when the two most powerful girls actively participated in cabin life. But, as camp progressed these two effectively withdrew from the group, thus leaving cabin power in the hands of two girls who abused it during the last week, resulting in an all-camp "scene" and eventually to their detention in the health clinic. Thus, a cabin group initially compatible ended in strife and disintegration when the power structure gradually eroded, completely breaking down during the last days of camp.

The Camp Session

The locus of attention in the cabin centered primarily with the Dinah-Gina duo, a relationship so intertwined as to make their impact as individuals secondary to consideration of them as a unit on the cabin. Of the two, Dinah was the ring leader, the creative motivator, inventor, and actor while Gina was the audience and the assistant.

From the outset until the last minute of camp the pair were seldom not in trouble, with cabinmates, cabin counselor, or the camp administration. Although at times Gina disapproved of the behavior and the "morality" of her best friend Dinah, her loyalty knew few limitations. With Dinah she could depend, with a fair degree of accuracy, on being a center of attention, a "someone" who had power and influence; she cared not that it was "negative" in nature. When Gina was not with Dinah she was liked by the other cabin members.

Dinah's humor was irritating to cabinmates; she would do almost anything for attention, for example, yelling obscenities at strangers passing by the cabin. It was nearly impossible to discipline her. Those from her home town who were at camp hardly acknowledged her presence. One junior counselor reported that Dinah apparently hated everyone, at least so it seemed to her. Another wrote that Dinah was the sole cause of the problems that she had with the cabin on DP's first day off. Once Dinah placed a penny under her tongue before going to the health clinic; the penny raised her body temperature, resulting in an excuse from swimming.

Dinah did not reciprocate Gina's friendship nomination, selecting Ava as her best friend. Of the 10 dyads in Cabin Seven, Dinah and Gina were involved in the most dominance encounters. Even though Dinah was the ring leader and Gina the audience, the latter dominated Dinah until the last 10 days of camp. When together during the first four weeks of camp Gina so readily followed that Dinah seldom initiated dominance over her. There were times when Gina countered Dinah; over one-quarter of her interactions with Dinah were refusals or shuns. She was considerably more indirect when dominating Dinah than Dinah was toward her.

By the end of the first week of camp the other three girls in the cabin complained to DP that Beth and Okie were taunted and ridiculed by Dinah and Gina. Ava was spared this teasing. They were resentful of the fact that they had to accommodate to the duo's time schedule, e.g., waiting for them at mealtimes and athletic activities.

Ava was the only cabin member "enthusiastic, powerful, and ornery enough to control Dinah," DP wrote after the second week of camp. But, by and large, she remained aloof from the daily cabin disputes even though she alone could unite the group. The other girls in the cabin, including Dinah and Gina, respected her opinions and judgments and followed her directives.

Ava selected Beth as her best friend because she most represented maturity, sensibility, and trustworthiness. The two seldom engaged in mutual dominance interactions. Ava was more dominant, primarily because Beth frequently recognized her superior status. Neither individual had a recorded instance of ridiculing the other.

Beth spent little time with the cabin group, preferring to be with a hometown friend who lived in another cabin. During the second week of camp her relationship with Gina became especially tense, even though she had earlier chosen Gina as her best friend. Later that week Beth was emotionally upset because "Gina and Dinah have been mean to me." They said that she called them "lesbians," and to get even with her they drew a picture of her and DP as siamese twins. During the first two-thirds of camp Beth dominated Gina and Dinah, primarily during cabin clean up. Gina was subordinated primarily by verbal directives and physical assertions; ridicule, however, was their most common mode of interacting. The Beth-Dinah dyadic level of interacting was the highest for both Beth and Dinah, and one of the most prevalent within the cabin. They frequently engaged in extended arguments that just lingered.

During the third week of camp Dinah and Gina increasingly solidified their partnership. When the cabin group went to the beach for a swim the pair walked together; on campouts they slept by themselves. Their ridicule of Oakie increased dramatically.

Originally, the group looked forward to Okie's slightly late arrival, and she was pleasant, talkative, and friendly, always wanting to tell someone what she did, was doing, or would do. Okie constantly did more than her share of the cabin work. One morning when the group was late for breakfast she told everyone to go; she would clean the cabin. During the first third of camp she was second only to Ava in her dominance success rate. But during the middle of camp her cheerfulness and happiness goaded Dinah and Gina, resulting in their dominance over her.

During the first two-thirds of camp Okie was either dominant over or equal in status with Gina and Dinah. But during the fourth and fifth weeks, this pattern was reversed as both Dinah and Gina increased their relentless countering and ridiculing behaviors over Okie. Without the former support of Ava and Beth, Okie fell from the beta to the omega position by the end of camp. Her former comrades tired of her "bubbliness" and "clinginess;" when she approached they shouted "Fly! Raid!" and giggled. Even though all cabin members were clearly dominating Okie, DP wrote at the end of the fourth week that she did not seem to care: "She is the calmest and the most cheerful." The episodes occurring during the last week (described below) ended this cheerfulness.

As the cabin situation became increasingly tumultuous during the middle of camp, Ava and Beth found extra-cabin friends as routes of escape; they disliked Dinah and Gina and rather than accept their ridicule as Okie did, they withdrew from association with the cabin group. Ava did not need cabin recognition for status and prestige; in fact, she was held in higher esteem when she associated with her older sister and her cabin. During the middle of camp her dominance success rate fell 20% and she reached her peak of non-participation in cabin dominance encounters. Beth apparently took her cue from Ava, escaping the cabin group to be with her hometown best friend. Her involvement in cabin dominance encounters declined almost 50% and her success dominance percentage dropped 20 points from the first to the last third of camp. During the last time period she did not dominate anyone in the cabin.

Gina reached her peak of dominance success during the middle third of camp, rising 21 percentage points as she dominated Ava in 50% of their interactions; Dinah's success percentage rose dramatically, from 28% to 53%, during the last third of camp. Only Ava was more dominant during the last time period. Paralleling this increase was a marked tendency for Dinah to be more overt when dominating others and for them to be more indirect when dominating her. The four girls responded to this rise in Dinah's status by doubling the number of recognition behaviors they had given to her during Time One and Time Two *combined.* For example, all of Gina's recognition of Dinah's superior status were initiated during the last 10 days of camp.

The brewing discontent reached its climax three days before the end of camp. DP walked into the cabin after "lights out" to find Okie shaking and crying; according to Okie, Dinah and Gina had been taunting her, throwing sand in her face, and playfully hitting her with a broom. They denied doing these things; Ava and Beth said nothing. The camp director came into the cabin the next day and admonished all for being "unnice." Dinah and Gina were furious, accusing DP of "blowing things out of proportion"—it was all done in fun.

Two days later Okie found a note on her bed entitled, "Things Wrong with Okie." Included in the list were such items as "doesn't share candy," "a nurd," and "counselor's pet." The list clearly implied that the writers hated her. When Dinah and Gina were confronted by the camp director, they vehemently denied writing it, that is, until the director told them that she had matched their application handwriting with the note. Neither Dinah nor Gina confessed until the director sentenced them to detention in the health cabin; Gina then said that it had been written in fun. Dinah chimed in that they had not intended for Okie to read it—"DP must have

put the note on Okie's bed in order to get us in trouble." Before going they
told DP how much they hated her, that it was all her fault, and that she
smelled like a dog. The two, however, refused to report to the clinic until
hours later when a camper friend, a cabin leader, and finally the security
guard persuaded them otherwise. That night the other girls of Cabin
Seven rearranged the beds for a peaceful evening of sleep.

The Data

It was basically a ridiculing group; one-third of all recorded dominance
behavior was verbal ridicule, significantly more than any other kind of
dominance behavior. There were no recorded instances of threat
behavior and only 10 observations of displacements and physical
assertions. Indirect expressions of dominance behavior were more
frequently observed than were overt strategies.

Although the overall frequency rate of recorded dominance behaviors
occurring per hour of observation time was relatively low, there was a
slight but nonsignificant increase in this rate over time. Daily fluctuations in the per hour occurrence of dominance behavior, highest during
the fourth and fifth weeks of camp when cabin crises were still brewing,
varied considerably. The average frequency rate quintupled during cabin
discussions but dropped 80% during mealtimes.

Considering data from the full camp session, seven of the 10 dyads
revealed a significant difference in directionality; two of the remaining
three approached significance. Ava significantly dominated all cabin
members; Beth dominated Gina and Dinah, but not Okie (approached
significance); Gina dominated Dinah but not Okie (approached significance); and Dinah and Okie evenly split their dominance interactions.
Dinah was placed ahead of Okie because of her domination over Okie
during the last third of camp.

Although a sigificant percentage of the dominance behavior occurring
during the camp was congruent with the dominance rank order, there
were frequent status shifts among the five girls. When the girls were
ranked during each time period there was a nonsignificant agreement
among the three orders. During the second and third time periods three
girls were tied for the middle three rankings. The girls ranked significantly the same on the indices of dominance; the reversal rate was only
significantly low during verbal directives.

The five girls also ranked significantly the same regardless of the
setting in which they were observed. Behavior occurring during rest hour
was not a reliable barometer of dominance relations, nearly one-half of
all dominance interactions observed during such times involved a
subordinate dominating a higher ranking individual.

On Day 3 when the girls rank ordered cabinmates on dominance, the
individual listings were not significantly intercorrelated. Beth was firmly

located in last and the other three girls were tied for first (Okie had not yet arrived). Nongroup observers did not rank order the five girls in such a way as to significantly agree with the behavioral dominance hierarchy. Three placed Dinah first and all underranked Beth. Most, however, placed Okie last.

A dominant girl in Cabin Seven was likely to be physically large, the least intelligent member of the cabin, and an ideal leader; the inverse held for low ranking girls. There was little tendency for an individual to interact most with those girls closest to her in the rank order—primarily because Dinah was everyone's most frequent dyadic partner—or for individuals high in dominance status to be the most actively involved in cabin dominance interactions. Three of the four best friend selections were individuals who ranked closest to the selector.

Conclusion

Dinah was the obvious choice for cabin mood setter, primarily because of her style of dominance. When she asserted herself, however, the others often contradicted, corrected, or ignored. During cabin discussions Dinah talked the most; but it was Ava's ideas that were acknowledged and accepted. When Ava declared her view, others nodded agreement. It was only Ava who united the cabin, essentially by effectively countering Dinah's influence.

Junior counselors who assumed leadership of the cabin on DP's days-off did not agree on who was the most dominant, Ava or Dinah. One wrote that Ava was a "sweet, nice, and quiet girl, too nice to be at the top of a dominance hierarchy." But another felt that Ava wielded considerable power among her peers; although Ava said little, she seemed to know everything. To these junior counselors Ava was dominant "in the right way" and Dinah, "in the wrong way."

The cabin, thus, had two dominant types within the group. Ava's prominence was indirect, she preferred giving directives and not arguing, ignoring, or countering. Her warmth, humor, and prestige solidified her prominence and power. Gina described Ava as the real "director of our group;" Dinah wrote that Ava is "nice and relaxed."

On the other hand, the group considered Dinah to be "icky, obnoxious, and messy." She was the most involved in dominance encounters, was one of the most overt, and dominated in the ways that Ava did not: arguing, ignoring, and countering. Dinah received 87% fewer recognition behaviors from group members than did Ava. When dominating her, cabin members were considerably more indirect than they were when they dominated Ava. Perhaps this reflects a fear of directly confronting Dinah. Indeed, the lower in rank, then the more likely one was to respond indirectly to Dinah.

Ava's response to Dinah and Gina was remarkably similar: ridiculing and directing. During cabin clean up Ava dominated the two in over 90% of their interactions. Nearly one-half of Ava's total dominance encounters were with Dinah; she was the only cabin member significantly dominated by Ava during all three time periods. But the two were more powerful than was Ava during counter dominance interactions.

Ava clearly recognized Dinah as her chief competitor for power in the cabin. But as Ava moved away from the group, and Beth followed her, a vacuum was left, filled by Dinah and Gina. With this development, primarily after the third week of camp, the cabin fell apart as the power structure within the cabin was inverted.

Cabin Eight

Overview

Despite the large number of personal conflicts, manifested by the unusually high frequency of psychosomatic illnesses, "unprovoked" cries, and initiated dominance acts, the five girls in Cabin Eight were consistent in the directionality of dominance behaviors occurring within the 10 dyads. Considered as a unit, they formed the basis for an almost rigid hierarchical ordering of the five girls. None of the five, however, reported at the end of camp that it was a pleasant summer; they did not enjoy the summer, but they did survive it.

For three of the five girls camp was a new experience; the other two, friends since the age of four years, were second year campers. These two set the tone for the summer; together they demonstrated shrewdness, charisma, manipulative skills, authoritative behavior, and peer prestige— all traits conducive to exerting and maintaining a firm control of power within the cabin.

The Camp Session

Alice and Barb controlled the mood, spirit, and power in Cabin Eight. Long time friends, during the first few days of camp they engaged in numerous water and pillow fights and made mockeries of serious cabin discussions by cracking dirty jokes or laughing at an "inside" joke. One evening when the other girls were playing "truth or dare" with JC, Alice and Barb came into the cabin and screamed, "Boy, are you guys queer!" The game ended. Cabinmates sought to be accepted by Alice and Barb, for the fun and for the status thus engendered. They were shuttled in and out of the winner's circle, depending on the whims of the pair.

But to other campers, leaders, and adminstrators, Alice and Barb were known as "double-trouble." From the first day of camp they were openly revolting and disobeying JC's cabin rules, as well as all-camp guidelines: quiet during rest hour, not swinging from the rafters, being on time for meals, etc. More so than Alice, Barb was the constant tester and antagonist of JC. The first day of camp she advertised her experience by boasting that she knew how to get around the requirements, and directly challenged JC by saying that she would not say any mealtime prayers because she was an atheist. She bragged that when drunk her father could beat up anybody; she was suspended from school for insulting teachers. Throughout camp Alice's power was indirectly wielded; when JC could not quiet the group during the first Sunday church service, Alice did so by refusing to respond to their play activity and by giving disapproving glances.

Even though each chose the other as "best friend," their relationship was somewhat tenuous during the first week of camp. Alice complained to JC that Barb was not doing her share of the work; the next day she announced to the cabin that she was not talking to Barb. The relationship was patched up by the next morning, but the friendship was never stable during the rest of camp. They interacted more frequently than did any other dyad in Cabin Eight, usually in an overt manner by direct orders. Alice was the dominant dyadic member during all three time periods, five behavior settings, and eight dominance indices of behavior. Barb favored Alice by warning the others in the mornings, "Let her sleep because she had a hard day yesterday." When Barb received a care package from home, only Alice was given the "special" flavor candy. She also made arrangements for Alice to meet a "cool" guy she knew from home—a secret meeting on the sand dunes.

By the end of the first week Deb was accepted into the "winners' circle," thus enhancing her assertion of dominance over a former rival, Ono. Deb's insecurity was readily apparent. When Alice told the cabin that her friends had given her a "going away to camp" party, Deb quickly asserted that her freinds too had a party for her—and over 1,000 people came! After several disbelieving looks she lowered the number several times. At school she was a body guard for a girl that she wanted to like her. Indeed, it was difficult not to "pick on" Deb; she almost seemed to want, even plead for it. JC wrote during the first week of camp:

Deb always places herself in a position of vulnerability and is, inevitably, always picked on. I just wish she could do something other than fear thinking about the fact that other people don't like her. She tries so hard to be liked. She'll do anything for a friend!

At Half-Christmas (June 25th) Deb made gifts for everyone in Cabin Eight; she most frequently sat beside Barb, Alice, and JC—the three highest status individuals in the cabin.

Deb willingly obeyed every directive of Alice and Barb, and during a Day 5 cabin discussion on goals for the summer, she repeated almost word for word what Alice and Barb had previously stated as their goals. On an overnight campout Deb offered to return to the cabin for a pillow that Alice said she wanted for that night's sleep. After Deb discovered that Barb refused to say meal prayers she too stopped saying them, preferring to rock back in her chair during grace—just like Barb. And just like Barb she, too, made paper airplanes during church services. One evening she wanted to skinny dip with Gladys, Ono, and JC, but Barb and Alice said it was "queer"; Deb decided not to go.

Alice and Barb's reaction to Deb was to treat her not as a mutual friend, but as a hand servant or play toy to tease and have fun with. Both dominated her in over 80% of their interactions with her, with neither setting, indice, nor time altering these one-sided relationships. In turn, Deb recognized their superior dominance status over six times as frequently as they recognized hers.

The differential treatment of cabin members by Deb is best illustrated by a Day 10 incident. On the sand dunes Deb jokingly called Gladys and Ono "lessies." The two joined forces with Alice and Barb to mummie-roll Deb into a blanket. But their fun ended when Deb panicked, screaming that she had sand in her eyes. Later, she apologized profusely to Alice and Barb for yelling at them—even though they were prepared to apologize to her—because she now "realized" that they had been trying to help her against the other two.

Once accepted by Alice and Barb, Deb became a "true believer," a blind follower unmerciful in criticism of underlings. Almost to the day that Deb was accepted into the Alice-Barb orbit, her subordination to Ono was reversed to domination, primarily by ridiculing and refusing to obey orders. Occasionally, her abuse became physical, one day hitting Ono twice in the mouth with the table cleaning sponge.

By the end of the first week, Ono told JC that she wanted to go home because the others, especially Barb, were ridiculing her by making faces, ignoring her when they said "goodnight" to each other, and not responding to her questions. Ono asked for food at the dinner table and no one would pass it. Or, she came into the cabin excited about something and no one would listen to her. Even though Ono could be just as vicious to others as they were to her, she could not physically nor mentally keep pace with her tormentors. By the middle of camp she no longer fought back, retreating to the periphery or physically attaching herself like a leach onto JC, babbling in babyishese to her "buddy buddy" cabin counselor. Ono was the only cabin member to wear the bracelet that JC made for everyone the first week of camp.

A swimming teacher told JC that the entire class disliked Ono. One day she had to rescue her from the deep water. Ono said later that she could not swim and had thus panicked; class members said it was a trick to get attention.

Gladys selected Alice as her best friend on the Day 4 sociometric, but it was not until the middle of camp that she was accepted by Alice as "cool." By the beginning of the third week Alice paired frequently with Gladys. The two seldom engaged in dominance interactions; Gladys became progressively more subordinate to Alice during the next five weeks. On a campout Alice and Gladys whispered and giggled for some time before going to sleep; Barb, the usual confidant in such secrets, was shunned. Several days later when Alice became ill she asked Gladys rather than Barb for emotional and practical (bring toothbrush) support. Barb, ignored by her ex-best friend, chummed with Deb.

With Alice's support Gladys became noticeably nastier toward Ono, increased her condemnation of Barb's antics, and challenged JC's authority. One evening she said "goodnight" to every cabin member, the cabin, the trees, the bugs, and, finally, to JC. During this middle third of camp Gladys achieved her highest dominance success percentage, especially increasing her domination over Deb and Ono. Yet, in a two-day period (Day 17 and 18) she was observed crying three times, due to a "cabin tenseness." Gladys reported ill to the health clinic, but the nurse discovered no physical cause for her "bellyache."

Thus, the net effect of the Alice-Gladys and the Barb-Deb alliances was to raise the dominance status of Gladys and to lower Deb's standing. The effect on the cabin group was to create an atmosphere of tenseness and chaos. One afternoon, during the third week of camp JC walked into the cabin to discover blankets hanging from the rafters that effectively partitioned the cabin into separate rooms. That evening, at the beach night supper there was little cooperation; no one picked up the food or agreed where to go for the campfire. As a result, supper was delayed and eaten in small groups and in shifts. This tenseness was also noted by junior counselors who stayed a hectic day with the group on JC's days off:

I had a distinct feeling of disunity—everyone did their job and only that one. Little bullying, everyone just seemed to be on the defensive. They were cooler, more aggressive, touchier, and less companionable than most cabins. It wasn't pleasant; it was pragmatic.

During the fourth week Ono, after being unmercifully ridiculed by Barb, reported "ill" to the health clinic, but she was released by the nurse when a source for her illness could not be found. When she came back to the cabin Barb sprayed her with Right Guard, to "protect" her against any more strange bugs. Earlier, Ono had selected Barb as her best friend. Now, she felt that only Gladys treated her decently, and the two were frequently observed to be sitting next to each other. But, after becoming "tight" with Alice, Gladys rejected Ono as "too much of a bad thing too often." Even though Gladys increased her dominance and ridicule, Ono never attempted to refute or counter her.

During the last week of camp, without warning or apparent reason, Alice suddenly shunned all in the cabin except Barb. The latter changed her mind about asking for a cabin switch, combining forces with Alice for a total domination of the group. "The silence" began. They refused to speak with anyone in the group, frequently laughing, ridiculing, and talking as if the others were not in the cabin; during rest hour they used a secret sign language. One day, Gladys became so upset that she stomped out of the cabin and refused to eat lunch because of "cabin tenseness." JC wrote, "The cabin has completely fallen apart, thanks to Alice and Barb."

Whatever cohesiveness existed previously was absent during the last week of camp. For example, Deb spent much time alone, staring at the beach or walking by herself. Her social alternative was to seek the friendship of those whom she had earlier ridiculed in her rise in dominance status. The Deb-Gladys relationship had always been tenuous, each using the other, until the last week when the dejected comrades found each other pleasant company.

"The silence" was primarily maintained by Alice; when she was not present Barb talked with the others, shutting up quickly if Alice appeared. What instigated Alice's behavior is somewhat mysterious. On Day 25 she went to the health infirmary with a bladder infection; the next day was JC's final day off. With Alice and JC "out of commission" Barb took over, exerting dominance over Gladys primarily through name calling and shunning, according to the junior counselor. Previous to this the two were equal in status, seldom engaging in dominance encounters. On Day 26 both JC and Alice returned to the cabin and "the silence" began. Alice demanded absolute allegiance from Barb and subordination from the others. Group dominance behavior changed from a 60% overt level to 60% indirect as Alice and Barb ignored, shunned, and talked about the others.

During the interval when Barb was shunned by Alice, she exhibited friendly behavior, saying grace at meals and calling JC by her first name. But once accepted by Alice, Barb resumed obstinancy, doing the opposite of what she was asked to do, openly challenging JC's authority, calling JC a "bitch" and a "Hitler," and running away when called. She told JC, "You're just here to keep us from killing each other."

Indicative of the disunity was the level of "cries" and "illnesses" during the camp session. In her notes JC wrote of 22 separate instances when one of the five girls cried. Gladys with eight and Deb with six were the most tearful, the two girls most frequently caught in the midst of power struggles. Reasons for crying varied: homesickness, intra-cabin squabbles, and physical pain. But the most common response was "won't tell."

Even more remarkable was the number of "psychosomatic" visits to the health clinic during the last two weeks of camp. Gladys complained of a "sick stomach"; Alice visited twice for an upset stomach, cramps, and a bladder infection; Deb and Ono had "hurt stomachs." The nurses were perplexed with Cabin Eight, suggesting to JC that the visits appeared to be psychologically and not physically induced. JC wrote: "So, as the cabin disintegrates, illnesses increase."

At the last Council Circle, a ceremony to symbolize the oneness of the camp and of the cabins, all five girls sat with friends from other cabins.

The Data

Verbal ridicule and recognition were the most frequently recorded indices of dominance status; four behaviors—physical assertion, verbal control, threat, and displacement—accounted for only 10% of the observed total.

Even though Cabin Eight had a high rate of dominance behavior (8.46 per hour), a large percentage was indirect (50%), frequently one girl recognizing the status of another. With such constant reminders of relative status position, the reversal rate was extremely low during all three time periods. There was no temporal increase or decrease in the frequency of dominance behavior observed, and fluctuations in the daily average of dominance behavior were not common. Four days during the first two weeks of camp were particularly volatile, due to special cabin activities: the friendship sociometric, two beach night suppers, and the first overnight campout.

Besides having the lowest reversal rate, mealtimes were also the behavior settings where dominance behavior was least likely to occur. Cabin activities had the highest frequency average.

All 10 dyads in Cabin Eight were significant and transitive in directionality; that is, Alice more frequently dominated the other four girls than they did her; Barb dominated Gladys, Deb, and Ono; Gladys, Deb and Ono; and Deb, Ono. Thus, the five girls can be ordered into a transitive dominance hierarchy, a rank ordering that remained essentially the same regardless of indice or setting.

The percentage of behavior transgressing a hierarchical arrangement of the girls (a Y dominating an X) was significantly less than behavior congruent with such a hierarchy. The reversal rate decreased as camp progressed, indicating a stabilization of dominance relationships over time. Two girls, Deb and Ono, reversed positions during the first week of camp; Barb and Gladys did not settle their relative status positions until the last week of camp.

After three days of camp, the girls rank ordered each other on relative dominance; the individual rankings were significantly correlated and significantly agreed with the Time One behaviorally derived dominance hierarchy. When the Cabin Seven leader (DP) ate lunch with the Cabin Eight girls during the second week of camp, her recorded dominance interactions were congruous with the behavioral rank order and the overall reversal rate. She and two junior counselors ranked the cabin on dominance; their listings significantly correlated with the behavioral hierarchy.

In Cabin Eight girls who ranked high on the dominance hierarchy were chronologically older, more intelligent, and more athletic than lower ranking group members. The higher in rank then the more apt was a girl to sleep far from the cabin counselor and to have other girls sit beside her. Best friends were not necessarily close in rank, but they did have their beds close to each other. The girls interacted in a dominance fashion most with those girls closest to them in the hierarchy.

Conclusion

The rigidity of the dominance group structure in Cabin Eight may be attributed to the fact that two very powerful, experienced campers who were best friends for over one-half of their lives were placed in the same cabin. Even though Alice and Barb controlled the interpersonal dynamics of the cabin, they were far from identical in their mode of exerting power. Alice was considerably more indirect when dominating and displayed more sympathy, until "the silence", in her interactions with the other girls. When Ono could not keep pace with the cabin on a hike, it was Alice who suggested that the group wait for her to catch up. On a Day 18 campout, Deb slightly injured her ankle. Alice became the "doctor," telling the others, "I know medicine." While Alice was the "director" of others, Barb was the "ridiculer." More so than Alice, Barb was the mood setter of the cabin, frequently telling dirty jokes. Her favorite was, "Why does Peter Pan fly? You'd fly too if your peter was hit by a pan!" During a game of charades she mimed a penis for the name "Dick Van Dyke."

The response of the other girls to them was also variable, giving nearly twice as many recognition behaviors to Alice than to Barb. They were more likely to sit beside Alice and to complain about Barb's behavior to JC.

One junior counselor wrote that Barb was the overt, aggressive, and dominant one while Alice was the creative idea that fed into and gave substance to Barb's antics. Even though both participated in "the silence," Barb seemed to derive a "demonic pleasure" in the havoc it wreaked on cabin unity—a sparse commodity.

6
Dominance Behaviors and Hierarchies in Male and Female Groups

The previous two chapters have provided a qualitative account of early adolescent interactions, more characteristic of anthropologists and ethologists than of psychologists. In the present chapter I count numbers, comparing the behaviors, group structures, and status characteristcs of the male and female adolescents in cabin groups One through Eight. A follow-up study, a questionnaire sent to the early adolescent boys several years after their camp session, and an all-camp study are described in the next section. An extended discussion focusing on a comparison of the sexes follows the presentation of the data.

Mode of Dominance Expression

Verbal ridicule was the most common and verbal/physical threats and object/spatial displacements were the least common expressions of dominance status among the young adolescents. There were some differences, however, between the sexes, as noted below (Table 6.1).

Boys were involved in considerably more physical play, fight encounters, and verbal arguments than were girls. But the most striking sex difference was in recognition of status behavior; giving compliments, asking favors, imitating, and soliciting advice occurred in every fourth encounter among female dyads, but only once in every 16 interactions among male dyads. Many of the female counselors noted this imitation in their observation notebooks, especially in regard to grooming, hair styling, and dressing; they were noticeably prevalent during the preparation time for the all-camp banquet and in the repetition of verbal cliches, such as "far out," "intense," and "I'm just weirded out." Boys also had their pet sayings, usually sexual in content (e.g., "You mo!"), but imitation seldom extended to other behaviors.

Regardless of the indice of behavior, girls were considerably more indirect when asserting their status than were boys; their 52% overtness ratio was substantially lower than the boys' 85%. The most overt female

TABLE 6.1

Female		Male	
ridicule	28%*	ridicule	27%*
recognition	23%	directives	19%
directives	22%	verbal control	15%
counter dominance	13%	physical assertion	15%
verbal control	7%	counter dominance	11%
physical assertion	5%	recognition	6%
threats	1%	displacement	4%
displacement	1%	threats	3%

*percent of total behavior observed for each indice for each sex.

cabin (57%) was less overt than the least overt male cabin (67%). As camp progressed girls became more indirect in exerting dominance, but boys became considerably more overt. By the last third of camp girls were more indirect than overt, 54%, and boys increased their overtness level to nearly 90%. Thus, during the last week of camp boys ordered, teased, argued, and physically asserted themselves while girls were more likely to be talking about each other, shunning, and giving unsolicited advice or information. The extreme form of this was manifested in Cabin Eight's "the silence," when two girls refused to speak to the other three during the last days of camp. In another group the two most dominant girls only talked to each other, but freely talked *about* the other three.

Frequency of Expression

During 402 hours of observations female groups averaged 6.34 instances of dominance interactions per hour; the male figures were 290 hours and 16.25 dominance interactions per hour. This large sex difference in frequency rate is further emphasized when the range for the female cabins—4.85 to 8.46—is compared with the male range—13.31 to 19.33.

But these results may be more artificial than real, for two reasons. First, as noted previously in the reliability checks, the female counselors were less likely to observe instances of dominance behavior than were male counselors. Second, and perhaps more pertinent, because girls are more indirect when expressing their dominance status, it is likely that more observations of female than male dyadic encounters were missed, or did not fit into the rather overt oriented indices of dominance behavior used in this study.

During the five weeks of camp the frequency rate in female groups *increased* but in male groups, with one exception, it *decreased* (Figure 6.1).

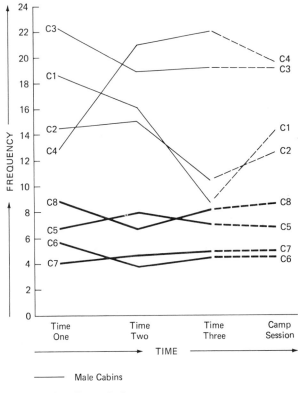

FIGURE 6.1

— — — Male Cabins

———— Female Cabins

Even though the frequency rate differential can be explained in part by reference to methodology, the temporal trend appears to be a basic sex difference.

Daily fluctuations in the per hour frequency rate of dominance behavior were considerably more common in female than male groups. Nearly 50% of all daily frequency rates in male cabins was within one-half of a normal distribution's standard deviation of the overall male per hour average of dominance interactions; only 30% of the female daily rates were within a comparable range of the overall female average. The wider spread of the female daily averages is further illustrated by the number of scores beyond one standard deviation of the sex's mean: 50% greater in female than in male groups (36% and 24%, respectively). Peak days of antagonistic encounters could usually be attributed to extra-curricular events in female groups, e.g., the formal banquet, campouts, beachnight suppers; but in male groups, more to internal contesting and squabbles than to external situational factors.

TABLE 6.2

Female		Male	
discussions	17.61*	activities	21.58*
activities	11.11	discussions	19.47
rest periods (bedtimes)	7.54	clean up/rest hour	18.86
clean up	6.46	rest periods (bedtimes)	16.76
mealtimes	2.90	mealtimes	10.93

*per hour frequency rate for each setting for each sex

In both male and female groups discussion and activity settings elicited the greatest frequency of dominance interactions. Mealtimes was a peaceful setting for all groups of early adolescents.

Dyads

Of the 82 intra-cabin dyadic combinations observed in the eight groups, 83% were significant ($p < .06$) in directionality (88% in females and 79% in males); another 6% approached significance. The 11% nonsignificant exceptions typically included a low ranking male who seldom interacted with other group members—the classical "loner."

In all eight cabins the reversal rate was significantly low,[1] ranging from 17% to 31% in female groups and 21% to 34% in male groups. That is, in all groups the higher ranking dyadic member dominanted the subordinate significantly more frequently than the reverse. Twenty-one of the 24 time period reversal rates were significantly low (11 in female and 10 in male groups).

In six cabins (three female and three male) the reversal rate decreased as camp progressed, indicating a stabilization of the dyadic dominance relationships over time. There were time shifts: 13% of the dyads flipflopped—an alteration in who was over the 50% mark in dominating the other—from one time period to another. In most cases these were statistically "undecided" dyadic relationships becoming directional.

The reasons for these shifts, as noted in the counselor's notebooks, would appear to be three:

1. a realignment of alliances or friendships within the cabin group, resulting in renewed challenges to the existing order

---

[1] Unless otherwise specified, significance implies the probability level is .05. "Approached significance" is reserved for instances when the probability level is between .06 and .15.

2. an individual troubled by personal issues withdrawing from inter-personal encounters
3. a new camper coming into the group and asserting himself or herself

Group Structure

Camp Session

Individuals in each cabin were linearly arranged into a dominance-submission hierarchy based on dyadic interactions. If individual A dominated B and B in turn dominated C, then in no case was C dominant over A. Because boys contested status relationships (higher reversal rates) more frequently, the girls were "easier" (fewer ties) to arrange into a hierarchy. The data are summarized for each cabin group in Appendix A.

These orders remained constant in seven of the eight cabins; that is, the three time period dominance hierarchies were significantly the same within a cabin. There were temporal shifts in status in all cabin groups, restricted primarily to single position changes (one up, one down). Several individuals, however, fell two places during the camp session. Most positional changes in the male cabins occurred among low ranking individuals. During each time period the first and second ranked boy maintained his hierarchical postion in all four cabins; however, four different ranked individuals during one time period or another in the four groups occupied the fourth and fifth slots. The most frequent shift in female groups was between the top two ranking girls, usually occurring during the second time period. The middle positions were least immune to permutations over time; at one time period or another individuals of all ranks occupied the second and third positions. With rare exceptions, once a female omega than always one, at least for the five weeks of camp.

Indices

In all cabins individuals ranked significantly the same regardless of the indice of dominance that was used to rank order them. Nearly 80% of all indice reversal rates was significantly low or approached significance (73% in female and 83% in male groups). The best predictors (low reversal rate) of dominance status were verbal directives and recognition of status behaviors, significantly low in seven and five groups, respectively; threat and displacement rates were significantly low in only two of the eight cabins.

Displacements and physical assertions were indicative of dominance position among males; however, in female groups these two indices

TABLE 6.3

Female		Male	
directives	18%*	recognition	19%*
ridicule	23%	directives	22%
threats	26%	displacements	24%
recognition	28%	threats	26%
counter dominance	30%	physical assertion	27%
verbal control	34%	ridicule	32%
physical assertion	35%	verbal control	36%
displacement	48%	counter dominance	39%

*average reversal rate for each sex for each indice of dominance behavior

frequently had high reversal rates. Ridicule was a considerably better predictor of status among females than it was among males. There was a clear relationship between frequency and low reversal rates in female dominance behavior: The most commonly expressed indicators of status were also the best predictors of the overall dominance hierarchy, in female but not male groups.

Setting

In all groups members ranked significantly the same regardless of the behavior setting in which they were observed. Ninety-two percent of all setting orders had reversal rates that were either significantly low or approached significance (84% in females; 95% in males). The reversal rate during cabin activities was significantly low in seven cabins; clean up behavior was the next best predictor of relative status.

In all male groups the discussion reversal rate was significantly low; in female groups, in only one. The best predictor of dominance position were those settings with the highest per hour frequency rate in male groups, but with the lowest in female groups.

TABLE 6.4

Female		Male	
clean up	20%*	activities	24%*
mealtimes	21%	rest periods (bedtimes)	27%
activities	24%	clean up/rest hour	28%
rest periods (bedtimes)	31%	discussions	29%
discussions	35%	mealtimes	29%

*average reversal rate for each sex for each behavioral setting

Sociometrics

When boys ranked cabinmates in terms of relative dominance status, six of eight times their individual listings were significantly correlated with each other. Aside from the two exceptions, which were rankings completed during the first week of camp, each sociometric composite cabin rank order was significantly correlated with the behavioral dominance hierarchy.

In two female cabins the group members' individual listings of dominance were significantly related; but in only one of these did the composite rank order significantly correlate with the behavioral dominance hierarchy.

Nongroup observers of the males accurately rank ordered the cabin under investigation nearly 90% of the time. This level of prediction was only 20% among nongroup observers of the female adolescents.

Characteristics

Few of the physical, behavioral, and social characteristics of individuals measured consistently predicted the group dominance hierarchy. Those that did, however, were basically the same for both sexes: athletic ability, pubertal maturity, and leadership. In addition, the most dominant boys were more indirect than were their subordinate cabinmates when dominating others and, as opposed to subordinates, dominant girls were more popular within the cabin group. The combined correlations and significance levels of various physical, behavioral and social characteristics with the dominance hierarchy are presented below (Table 6.5).[2]

Several differences between the sexes are apparent. Popularity among peers and chronological age were more predictive of status in female than in male groups. On the other hand, dominant boys were more physically attractive and of higher socioeconomic rank than were lower ranked boys; those were not characteristic of female groups.

When asked to place themselves in their group's dominance hierarchy, young adolescents more frequently perceived themselves as higher in rank than cabinmates placed them (36% and 21%). In more cases, however, the two placements were the same (44%). Boys more so than girls accurately perceived their rank (55% and 33%); girls were more likely to underrank themselves (28% and 13%).

There was relatively little relationship between dominance status and camp experience, or between how much the counselors liked the youth

---

[2] To test the significance of combined results, a chi-square transformation was performed that tests the hypothesis that the composite "p" value for the several findings could have occurred by chance (Jones & Fiske, 1953).

TABLE 6.5

Characteristic	Females		Males	
	Correlations	P Values	Correlations	P Values
Leadership	.82	.05	.92	.00
Athletic ability	.56	.05	.60	.05
Pubertal maturation	.55	.10	.59	.05
Physical fitness	—	—[a]	.66	.05
Overtness	−.30	ns	−.57	.10
Popularity (early)	.63	.10	.22	ns
Sit beside	.65	.10	—	—[a]
Physical size	.28	ns	.37	ns
Intelligence	.30	ns	.37	ns
Bed position	−.51	ns	.08	ns
Hiking order	—	—[a]	.54	ns
Socioeconomic status	−.10	ns	.41	ns
Attractiveness	.01	ns	.46	ns
Counselor's favorites	.18	ns	.29	ns
Chronological age	.33	ns	.03	ns
Socioempathy of rank	−.27	ns	.08	ns
Popularity (late)	—	—[a]	.32	ns
Involvement	.03	ns	.07	ns
Creativity	—	—[a]	−.03	ns

[a]Not measured.

and his or her dominance rank. Intelligence, creativity, empathy, age, physical attractiveness, and physical size were also relatively unimportant in predicting status among these adolescents.

The relationship between dominance rank and sibling order is suggestive but incomplete. Of the 40 early adolescents in the study none are "only" children; nearly 50% are, however, the youngest in their family. In every case, the top ranked female is the youngest child in the family and the last ranked girl, the oldest. Males neither countered nor supported these findings.

Nearly 80% of the best friend selections was with individuals ranked adjacent to the selector, twice the rate expected by chance. Best friends also tended to sleep closest together (expected/E: 25%; observed/O: 51%), but they were an unstable commodity as 50% of all such selections changed from the first to last week of camp.

It seemed reasonable to expect neighboring ranked individuals to interact more with each other in dominance encounters—because of status competition—than with any other ranked individual. This expectation was not supported by the data (E: 39%; O: 48%); neither did the youths interact most with the first (E: 32%; O: 24%) nor last (E: 32%; O: 34%) best friends. In all of these relationships there was no notable sex difference.

Styles of Dominance and Submission

Within the female and male groups there were similarities among individuals in their style of dominance behavior toward others and in their physical, behavioral, and social characteristics. Although this is not a rigid specific type × rank typology, it does answer those (e.g., Bernstein, 1981) who argue for commonalities in characteristics existing across groups of "Nth" ranked individuals—other than the top and bottom ranked individuals (see Chapter 10 for discussion of alphas and omegas). Not all "types" were represented in each cabin; neither did all cabins have only one of each type. Some individuals did not fit into any of the listed classifications. (Cabin numbers are in parentheses.)

Males

Peer Leaders Alan (One), Ara (Two), and Alex (Three) were "peer leaders," frequent initiators of verbal directives and most successful when displacing cabinmates. More than any other cabin member, leaders were indirect when initiating dominance. During the camp session they became less involved in dominance interactions, but others still frequently recognized their superior status. In athletic games peer leaders were the cabin member most likely to assert dominance; during cabin discussions their ideas received the most votes as over 50% of all suggestions they made was accepted by the group.

Although peer leaders were not necessarily the oldest, the most pubertally advanced, or the largest boy in the cabin, they were above the group average on these three dimensions. In all cases each was the best athlete in the cabin, demonstrating a finesse and coordination lacking in most agemates. They were judged to be the most handsome and one of the most intelligent boys in the group. Cabinmates described peer leaders as dominant, rich, handsome, athletic, popular, stubborn, and strong and as the leader and cabin bully. They were also liked by the cabin counselor. A peer leader's family was wealthy and usually contained younger brothers.

Bullies "Bullies" Gary (One), Gene (Two), and Andy (Four) were most successful asserting their status by threats or physically oriented behaviors. But, during verbal exchanges such as verbal control and ridicule and during discussions, they were as likely to be subordinate as dominant. A bully overrated himself on the dominance sociometrics and described himself as being more positive—handsome, masculine, smart, and strong—than peers portrayed him: stubborn, loud, and bullish.

For their chronological age bullies were physically mature, being the tallest and heaviest member of the group, but also the youngest; thus, bullies were early maturers. Despite their size advantage, bullies were rated as average athletes. All have large families that include an older sister. Cabinmates frequently expressed regret that such individuals were in the cabin; bullies usually ranked last on the friendship sociometrics.

Jokers Bobby (One), Doug (Two), and Eric (Three) were the cabin "jokers," most successfully dominant when verbally ridiculing cabinmates, especially at mealtimes. During athletic contests jokers were more often subordinate than dominant. They were considered by peers to possess leadership skills that were seldom behaviorally used and to be funny, friendly, and dumb.

Although they were the same age as peer leaders, jokers were more than two years less pubertally mature. Despite being the shortest and lightest cabin member, they were one of the best athletes in the group. Jokers enjoyed peer popularity; cabin counselors were not so highly appreciative of them. A middle child in a large and wealthy family, all jokers have a younger sister.

Quiet Followers During one time period of camp, Don (One), Ed (One), Ernie (Two), and Delvin (Four) were omegas, rising a postion or two before the end of camp. Infrequent participants in cabin dominance interactions, these "quiet followers" were most successful when expressing counter dominance; they were least dominant when giving directives. Cabinmates described them as mature, quiet, and dumb.

Quiet followers were the oldest member of their group, but pubertally they were average in timing. Short, light weight, uncoordinated, and physically unattractive, quiet followers were not popular among peers, becoming even less so as camp progressed.

Submissive Followers The four omega ranked boys—Oscar (One), Omar (Two), Orville (Three), and Otto (Four)—were "submissive followers." During cabin discussions their ideas were frequently ignored or ridiculed. Others seldom recognized their status, successfully dominating them by physical or verbal threats but not by verbal arguments. Cabinmates described submissive followers as weak, submissive, poor, friendly, and religious, and the submissive followers agreed with this assessment.

Submissive followers were late maturers, almost childlike. They were either chronologically young or a first year camper. Although not necessarily short in height, most were light weights, physically unfit, and weak; all ranked last in their cabin group on athletic ability. With one exception, their family was from a lower socioeconomic status than most other cabin members' family. Submissive followers were average in the cabin on handsomeness, popularity, dominance involvement, and overtness.

Females

Maternal Leaders Amy (Five), Ann (Six), Ava (Seven), and Alice (Eight) were "maternal leaders." Frequently indirect, they gave unsolicited advice on proper dress, manners, and grooming. They were perceived by peers as a source of security and support and were described as confident, loyal, kind-hearted, and manipulative.

They were pubertally mature, physically large, and chronologically old in comparison to cabinmates. Liked by both peers and adults, maternal leaders demonstrated intelligent behavior and ideal leadership traits. Within their family, they were the youngest child.

Antagonists Betty (Five), Becky (Six), Gina (Seven), Dinah (Seven), and Barb (Eight) were the "antagonists" in the female groups. They were the most actively involved in cabin dominance encounters, frequently countering or refuting cabinmates; they were not successful, however, in dominating others by verbal directives or arguments. Cabinmates frequently recognized their superior status position. Described by counselors as mood setters, antagonists were overt when dominating others. They were portrayed by peers and adults alike as assertive, aggressive girls who imposed themselves on others, enticing other girls to join them in breaking camp regulations; as charismatic, spirited individuals; and as problem campers who possessed negative leadership characteristics and who continually contested the authority of the counselor.

In every female group the best athlete was an antagonist and she was also one of the most physically mature. The antagonist was always a returning camper, coming from a wealthy, but not necessarily stable family. All have older brothers and are one of the youngest in their family. After an initial attraction, an antagonistic girl usually lost her peer popularity as camp progressed. Not unexpectedly, she was frequently the cabin member least appreciated by the counselor.

Amorphous Miss Average Four girls can be characterized as possessing "amorphous miss average" traits: Donna (Five), Gloria (Six), Beth (Seven), and Gladys (Eight). Their distinguishing pattern was the lack of one—average in most indices and settings in their use of and success at dominance behaviors. Usually the least involved in dominance inter- actions, as camp progressed they fell in dominance success. Cabinmates described them as non-descript, placid, shy, quiet, neat, "just there," and "the most forgettable character."

Despite being one of the youngest members of the cabin, miss averages were usually the tallest and the heaviest. On most other characteristics, however, they were average. Three of the four were first year campers, all have large families and many sisters, and all were liked by their cabin counselors. Cabinmates perceived the amorphous girls as having a potential for leadership that was not manifested behaviorally.

Compliant Clingers The "compliant clingers" included Olivia (Five), Dottie (Six), Opal (Six), Okie (Seven), Deb (Eight), and Ono (Eight). These girls frequently recognized the superior dominance status of cabinmates by giving favors and compliments. When dominant, a rare event, they usually engaged in verbal arguments. Compliant clingers apparently set themselves up for being picked on, an almost universal reaction to them. This vulnerability was most obvious in their tendency to constantly monitor surrounds. Cabinmates described this type of girl as friendly, talkative, and extroverted; however, they avoided her, considering her an embarrassment. If shown attention, the compliant clinger physically held on like a "leech."

Compliant clingers were the worse athletes, the most pubertally immature, the shortest, and the lightest. In most cases each was the oldest child in a wealthy family. Four of the six were first year campers. They possessed few leadership traits, were not popular with peers, and slept closest to the cabin counselor.

Conclusion

Male Cabins

Cabins Two and Three were cohesive groups throughout the camp session; One and Four only became compatible during the last week of camp after resolving several interpersonal conflicts.

Of the four, the group structure in Cabin One was the most adhered to—no other cabin had such uniformly low reversal rates in the eight indices, five behavior settings, and three time periods. The frequency rate, which fluctuated widely from day to day, dropped 50% as camp progressed. Cabin One was the only group in which the most dominant members, as opposed to low ranking boys, were also the most frequently involved in dominance encounters.

The Cabin Two hierarchy was extremely visible to the group members, as ascertained in their behavior and sociometric placements. No other cabin group had such a high proportion of overt forms of dominance behaviors, or had a lower frequency rate.

The boys in Cabin Three were a full year younger than the other boys in the study. In comparison to the other groups, they had the lowest overt ratio, reversal rate, and daily fluctuation level in frequency rate. Verbal directives, rather than ridicule, was the most frequently expressed form of dominance behavior, especially in regard to giving unsolicited advice. No other alpha experienced such a high level of dominance success; his "maternalistic" behavior heavily colored all cabin interactions. Physical assertions and physical/verbal threats were seldom observed.

No other cabin group had a greater number of physical assertiveness encounters, nor, more specifically, had so many serious physical fights as did Cabin Four. Still, over 90% of all physical assertions were play fights. The alpha and omega individuals were not typical in that the former was not a peer leader but a bully and the latter was more assertive than most other last rank boys. The reversal rate was higher than in any other male cabin, becoming significantly low only during the last third of camp. The frequency rate, the highest of any cabin group, significantly increased as camp progressed.

Apparently, neither a transitive, tightly organized (One) nor a loose, intransitive (Four) dominance hierarchy is necessary for interpersonal compatibility and group stability. In the former, the frequency of dominance behavior was considerably below that of the latter, but both were problematic cabin groups. Compatibility in Cabin Two and Three was achieved in quite different manners: visible (Two) versus discrete (Three) recognition of the dominance hierarchy; overt (Two) versus indirect (Three) behavioral strategy patterns; and low (Two) versus high (Three) frequency rate. In both, the group dominance hierarchy was well formed, yet flexible in that some movement among group members occurred; however, the reversal rate was always significantly low.

Female Cabins

The four female groups were both unique and similar in their dominance behavior and structural patterns. Cabins Five and Six were apparently the cohesive groups while Seven and Eight were both fraught with severe interpersonal conflicts.

Cabin Five was the only group to cry together at the closing ceremony. Even though the highest ranking girls were the most indirect in dominating others—the only cabin with such a pattern—as a total group they were the most overt females in their dominance strategies. The hierarchy was not rigid; as camp progressed the reversal rate increased slightly and there were fluctuations among the middle ranking girls. Relative to the other cabin groups, compliments were rare but threats were comparatively common.

Despite the fact that Cabin Six girls were one year older (14.3 years) that the others, on almost every dimension they were in the middle of the four groups. For example, they varied less from the female average on percentage usage of the various sub-categories of dominance behavior than did any other group.

Of the four, Cabin Seven had the least stable dominance hierarchy: The three time period orders were not significantly related; the reversal rate was the highest of the four groups; the indice rankings were barely significantly intercorrelated; few of the physical, behavioral, or social dimensions predicted the dominance hierarchy; neither the girls nor nongroup observers accurately rank ordered the group; and daily fluctuations from the overall behavioral frequency rate were greater than in any other cabin. The girls of Cabin Seven were the most indirect when dominating each other, with a frequency rate lower than any other female group.

Cabin Eight's pattern was a rigid hierarchy with a high but consistent frequency rate of dominance behavior. Although counter dominance behavior was not an accurate predictor of status in the other three female cabins, it was highly indicative of relative dominance in Cabin Eight. The group was also unique in being the only cabin in which the maternal and antagonistic girls were best friends and collaborators. In the other three cabins the two girls did not work together, usually ignoring the other as much as possible. The effect of collaboration was to allow the two girls in Cabin Eight to gain a firm hold of cabin power, usurping authority from the cabin counselor and preventing underlings from gaining any power base. The result was an inflexible dominance hierarchy, a high frequency of conflictual behaviors, and a large number of both direct conflicts (cries) and psychosomatic complaints (illnesses).

Even though Cabin Seven and Eight were alike in that both experienced chaotic last week events—"the detention" and "the silence"—they were in many respects opposite: high (Seven) versus low (Eight) reversal rates; low (Seven) versus high (Eight) frequency rates; and high (Seven) versus low (Eight) daily fluctuations in dominance behavior. In Cabin Seven the maternal and antagonistic girls ignored each other (24 interactions), whereas these two girls in Cabin Eight were mutually involved in 133 dominance encounters.

Apparently, neither a tightly (Eight) nor a loosely (Seven) ordered dominance hierarchy is conducive to group stability. The most unified cabins, Five and Six, were the only ones with a relatively stable and yet flexible dominance structure.

All Cabins

Various factors can be attributed to account for the cohesiveness of young adolescent groups: the personality of group members, the leadership style of the cabin counselor, and chance happenings ("fate"). The most cohesive groups in the present study had a relatively stable and yet flexible dominance structure. Neither a rigid, ordered nor a loose, transient dominance hierarchy was characteristic of united and harmonious groups. Whether the group structure determines group unity or the compatibility of group members dictates the structure is not discernible from the data provided by the eight cabins; they only indicate that the two are related.

Extended Studies of Dominance

The first study described below explores the centrality of dominance status in the lives of the early adolescent boys by asking each to recall the dominance position of all members of his former camp group. A number of ethologists (Bernstein, 1981; Chalmers, 1981; Seyfarth, 1981; Smuts, 1981) have questioned the stability of dominance rank over time within the same group of individuals. In the second study data collection from boys of all ages attending Camp Wancaooah during the first and third data years at camp are reported. Thus, research questions requiring a data base far larger than individual cabin groups and including a wider age range are addressed.

Recall of Dominance Status

Six months after the data from Cabins Three and Four were collected in Boys Camp, a questionnaire postcard was sent to the participants in the pilot study, Cabin One, and Cabin Two. This represents a time span of 3½, 2½, and 1½ years, respectively. The boys were asked to "List the campers in your (year) cabin, including yourself, in order of dominance. Remember the way it was then: Who exerted the most power or influence and who got his own way?"

All 18 boys returned the postcard. Intra-group agreement in the three groups were as high or higher than their end of camp dominance ordering years earlier.[3] The three after-camp dominance hierarchies were significantly correlated with their counterparts at the end of the camp session.[4] The boys most remembered who the alpha (17 of 18) and beta (14 of 18) individuals were.

All-Camp Study

Study One Methods. There were 32 cabin groups at Wancaooah Boys Camp during the pilot study summer. During a last week group session each boy was asked by his cabin counselor to rank group members on dominance and friendship as defined elsewhere in this book. Of the eight "A" cabins (10-11 year olds), three (17 individuals) completed this exercise; of the eight "B" cabins (11-12 year olds), six (35 individuals); of the eight "C" cabins (12-13 year olds), seven (39 individuals); and of the eight "D" cabins (13-15 year olds), seven (40 individuals). Thus, 23 groups (72% of the 32 total) and 131 boys (71% of the 185 total) participated in this project.

The 32 cabin counselors were asked to rank their group on dominance, pubertal maturation, athletic ability, and mental ability. All completed this task during the last week of camp.

Study Two Methods. Two summers later all boys at Camp Wancaooah were asked to complete the dominance sociometric. In group sessions

---

[3] Xr^2's = 24.10, 21.52, and 26.38; all $ps < .01$.
[4] r's = .94, .68, and .92; $ps < .01$, .08, and .01, respectively.

conducted by the cabin counselors, 31 of the 32 groups completed the rank ordering. This represents 96% (145 of 151) of the boys in camp.

All 32 cabin counselors rank ordered their group on dominance. In addition, they were asked to designate youths who were "problems" in the group.

Study One and Two Results

1. Do the boys agree among themselves on the relative dominance rank of their group?

    Of the 52 cabin groups in the two years (two groups had only three boys in them and so are omitted from further analysis), 45 or 87% agreed among themselves on the relative dominance rank order of the group.[5] Of the remaining seven, four were significant at the .10 level. Thus, the answer is an overwhelming "yes."

2. Do the cabin counselors agree with their group's dominance ranking?

    In 26 of the 52 groups (50%) the cabin counselor agreed with the dominance hierarchy from the boys' rankings with correlations ranging from an average of .59 to .93 in the four age groups. The average correlation for all 52 groups is .76, which is highly significant. The cabin counselors were apparently aware of the group hierarchy, but not as aware of it as were the boys.

3. Did the cabin counselors' assessments of the boys' relative pubertal maturation, athletic ability, and mental ability agree with the group's derived dominance hierarchy?

    Athletic ability (mean correlation was .71 with a range in individual cabins of −.23 to 1.00) was highly related to the group dominance hierarchy. Less predictive were pubertal maturation with a mean correlation of .35 (range = −.43 to .90) and mental ability with a mean correlation of .14 (range = −.50 to .70).

4. Is one's dominance and friendship status similar?

    There was a strong indication (mean correlation of .54; range, −.20 to 1.00) that the most dominant boys were also the best liked by their peers.

5. Which boys are most likely to cause "problems" in the cabin? Who are the most likely to return the following summer to camp?

    The cabin counselors noted the names of 42 "problem" campers. The most frequently (58%) listed were second or last ranked boys. Alphas were seldom labeled as problem boys.

    Beta ranked boys were also the most likely to return to camp (72%). Next most likely were omegas (56%). Alphas (32%) and middle ranked campers (46%) were least likely to return to camp. Thus, the problem youths were most likely to return to camp the following summer.

---

[5] Xr^2s = 8.70 to 28.95, all $ps < .05$.

6. Does a returning camper have a higher dominance rank than a new camper?

Of the 15 individuals who returned to camp from Study One to Study Two (two years), nine rose one or more places in the hierarchy, four remained the same, and two went down in rank.

Comparing the mean rank of 144 returning campers with the mean rank of 81 first time campers (unknown = 51) revealed the former to be significantly higher in rank than the latter.[6] Of 42 alphas, 30 (71%) were returning campers (expect by chance: 64%).

Thus, camp experience was beneficial, but certainly not the major contributor to one's dominance rank.

7. What are the major differences between alpha and omega ranked boys?

As ranked by their cabin counselors, alphas were more athletic and pubertally mature, but not more intelligent. Peers rated alphas as better liked.[7]

8. When the boys ranked their group on dominance, what status positions were most obvious to group members? Who was the most likely to be accurate in self-assessment?

At all age levels there was greatest agreement on the alpha (76%) and omega (66%) positions. Mid-ranked boys were less frequently accurately placed (41%).

Alpha and beta ranked boys were most accurate in assessing their relative self rank (67% and 68%, respectively). Middle ranked boys were more likely to overrank themselves (74%) than to be accurate (23%). Of the 276 campers, 46% were accurate in their dominance self-assessment (agreed with the group's placement of them); 43% over-ranked themselves and 11% underranked themselves.

9. In all of the above questions, are their age trends?

Spanning the years 11 to 15, there were relatively few age trends. During pre- or early adolescence (A cabins), however, pubertal maturation was a much stronger predictor of dominance status than it was during middle adolescence (D cabins) (correlations of .60 and .27, respectively). With increasing age mental ability became a better predictor of dominance rank (correlations from .07 to .31).

Female Groups

The manner in which an adolescent girl behaves with peers in natural contexts, her everyday world, has seldom been a primary research interest of social or behavioral scientists. Despite the empirical disinterest,

---

[6] $t = 2.86, p < .005$.
[7] $t = 11.12, p < .000; t = 5.67, p < .000; t = .62, NS; t = 4.64, p < .000$.

theoretically, many have argued that relations with peers become a crucial developmental task of adolescence if "normal" social development is to proceed (see reviews in Savin-Williams, 1980b, and Hartup, 1983). But there is an expanding literature (e.g., Gilligan, 1982; Holstein, 1976; Small, 1984) that illustrates that one cannot simply generalize from studies of males to the behaviors, psychological processes, cognitive abilities, and group structure of females among human and nonhuman primates.

Several investigations have reported on the natural behavior of adolescent females. M. Mead (1928) based *Coming of Age in Samoa* on observations of adolescent girls in the natural surroundings of Samoan culture and social settings. In *Elmtown's Youth*, Hollingshead (1949) was with adolescents "whenever and wherever possible" to discover the experiences of individuals within the social contexts of both the peer group and the larger community. These early naturalistic studies of adolescent females, however, were based on data that were more impressionistic accounts of female behavior than they were quantifiable recordings of behavior.

Sherif, Kelly, Rodgers, Sarup, and Tittler (1973) observed informal groups (N's=6-7) of girls over a 14-month period of time at a high school. Seven natural groups were identified based on frequent and recurrent patterns of interaction. Sherif et al. reported on (1) group labels (e.g., wild ones, long hairs, sports, rurals) based on an observer's perception of normative concerns; (2) group cohesiveness; and (3) role structures, especially in regard to high and low status individuals. These observational findings, however, were a reflection of the observer's impressions and not based on data that were subjected to statistical analysis.

Weisfeld, Weisfeld, and Callaghan (1982), on the other hand, used their observational data of girls in natural settings to note actual behavior interactions. Both direct observations and film were employed to assess sex differences in playground competition during dodgeball games. Although the methodology corrected a major research shortcoming of peer relations among girls, the focus of the research did not examine the internal structure of female groups—the major concern in this volume.

In my earlier review of adolescent females in natural groups (Savin-Williams, 1980b), four conclusions about female groups were drawn: (1) Females are less likely than males to form a stable and consistent peer group; (2) female groups are likely to be cliquish and relatively small (i.e., pairs or threesomes as opposed to male gangs); (3) a female group is likely to be less structured than a male group, though a definite leader is recognized behaviorally if not verbally; and (4) the group aids females in developing socioemotional, interpersonal skills and sensitivities. Meek's study (1940) found that although 7th grade girls value popularity with all groups, it is more important to a 12th grade girl to be accepted by a small select clique and to have one special friend for emotional support. By late adolescence female friendships are stabilized, and much of the bickering, jealousy and rivalry commonly reported in female early adolescence wanes (Meek, 1940). M. Mead (1928), in her study of Samoan girls, also found that 16- and 17-year-old girls congregate "in groupings of twos and threes, never more" (p. 67). Douvan and Adelson (1966) viewed an all-female group as "a source of narcissistic supplies" for a girl and stated that the solidarity of a peer group is much more important to boys than it is to girls.

It is rare that the concept of dominance hierarchy or any other "power" structure is used in reference to female groups, either among human or nonhuman primates. Although some recognize that certain female adolescents stand out as most influential or as a leader, there is considerable disagreement as to the characteristics of adolescent female group leaders. From his questionnaire data, Coleman (1961) concluded that the following were of primary importance for leading crowd girls: good personality, good looks, well dressed, and successful relationships with boys. Hollingshead (1949) found careful grooming, proper language, and social class important characteristics of leaders of both sexes, and for girls a good sexual reputation was also important. In a recent study Weisfeld, Bloch, and Ivers (1984) reported that boys strive for social success primarily through competence in athletics; girls achieve status through cultivating an attractive appearance. Dominant girls were perceived by peers as fashionable, attractive, and well-groomed.

Camp Wancaooah Adolescents

Group Geist

Among adolescents at Camp Wancaooah the two sexes diverged considerably in their manifestation of dominance behavior. Although there were severe interpersonal conflicts in cabin groups from Day 1, a polite stage at the beginning of camp was evident in both sexes of early adolescents. But, boys were "nice" to each other for only a few short days before full scale conflict developed. Girls, however, were polite to each other for several more days, often to the consternation of their counselors who deplored the lack of genuine relations during the first week.

Male dyads experienced conflict more quickly, frequently, and overtly than did female pairs. Although this is supported by the empirical data, there is another element that more clearly separates the two sexes: The conflict among boys can best be described as "mean" and among girls, as "vicious" or "cruel." All four female counselors felt this cruelty in their group; they hated it and tried to change it, but were to the woman unsuccessful. At one point or another all four said that the conflict was so prevasive and uncontrollable that they cried or wanted to go home.

Conflict among boys was potentially physically injurious (towel flipping at buttocks or groin area, wrestling, and throwing eggs, oranges, peanut butter, etc.), but short-term. Grudges were rare because attempts to reconcile differences, or at least to tolerate them, after physical fights or verbal arguments were made.

All male groups made a concerted and successful attempt to resolve the major interpersonal conflicts during the last weeks of camp. Only one of the female groups touched a resolution stage; in the others, interpersonal conflicts appeared to multiply and not decrease over time. Whether the girls were incapable of resolving conflicts or were unable or unwilling was not clear. One of the female counselors wrote in her journal, "The girls did not get along because they were not suffering together; they did not seem to need each other as most cabin activities did not emphasize cabin unity. Rather, status cliques based on popularity, beauty, athletics, and sociability were the important social unit." Another agreed, "Basically, I had a horrible and miserable summer, topped by the last days of camp. But, it seemed to be a bad summer for many. There was not much cabin spirit as the cabin mood changed so much from day to day. I saw much split allegiances with few girls seeing any reason to make the cabin work. Most did not give a damn about their tribe or their cabin group; they just did not care."

Dominance Behaviors

Boys were more likely to physically assert themselves, argue with others, and, to a lesser extent, verbally or physically threaten and displace cabinmates; girls were more likely to recognize the status of others, give unsolicited advice and information, shun, and ignore. Although these sex differences in behavior may be most obvious in violent (criminal), aggressive, or competitive encounters (Ramirez & Mendoza, 1984; Wilson & Daly, 1985), they are also evident in helping behavior (Chapter 8): Girls were three times more likely than boys to verbally help a group member and boys were three times more likely than girls to physically assist another. This reflects the general trend for boys to be direct and girls to be indirect in interpersonal encounters. Young adolescent males thus *asserted* their status through the "power" related components of dominance behavior; girls *expressed* their status through evaluative behavior.

Kaplan's work (1971) suggests that the discrepancy in many studies of sex differences in power, authority, and leadership may be due to the criteria employed to assess dominance. Although toughness and physical aggression measures will usually place most boys at a higher rank than most girls, other tasks such as picture drawing, personal closeness, and verbal behavior, will elicit no sex differences in dominance. Or, as Maccoby and Jacklin (1974) assert, perhaps power rank does not generalize to situations where aggression is not appropriate. Wilson and Daly (1985) document the "dangerous-young-male syndrome" in crime statistics; female adolescents also take risks and compete but they are less intense and less physical.

Cronin (1975) substantiates these views. Boys were usually nominated by peers as the toughest (84% of all nominations were boys); girls achieved social prominence by placing high on the "most grown-up" sociometric (82% of all nominations were girls). Opal, the girl who ranked highest on this dimension, dominated the female group whenever they played together, and she was the girl most likely to participate in male activities.

In the early adolescent studies, as the camp session progressed most male dyads decreased their frequency, but increased the overtness level of dominance encounters. This supports the position that a hierarchical arrangement of group members abets antagonistic interactions, thus enhancing the prospects for group order and harmony. The female pattern was of a different nature and thus, perhaps, had different effects. Rather than reducing the frequency and raising the overtness of dominance relations, female dyads tended to increase the frequency rate and to have less visible and more indirect interactions.

The female pattern of expressing altruism and recognizing authority in an indirect, verbal fashion is considerably more conducive to developing and maintaining close knit relationships than is the more competitive and direct assertion of power by males. In the camp studies, the adolescent females varied this frequency rate of dominance interactions in accordance to the situation. This indicates their greater willingness to accommodate behavior to the particular activity, implying a greater sensitivity to the surrounds and to the complexity of the social environment. Male status seldom changed; fluctuations in the dominance hierarchy occurred primarily among the followers. An alpha girl during the middle of camp often slipped to the beta position before regaining her prominence during the last week of camp. There is female flexibility, temporally as well as situationally.

Group Structure

The female age extension research reported in the next chapter as well as particular trends among the early adolescent girls (sharing power among the top two ranking girls) raise doubts that the dominance hierarchical structure so prevalent in male adolescent groups is adequate to describe status differentiation among adolescent females. Although the quantified data indicate that the female adolescent interactions could be construed on a group level as a dominance hierarchy, the ethnographic data described in Chapter 5 leave little doubt that a linear, stable hierarchy did not exist in any female group, except Cabin Eight. This latter conclusion should not be surprising because among many nonhuman primate species, adolescent females seldom congregate in groups; when they do, they are more likely to form cliques of twos or threes than form dominance hierarchies in relative larger groups (Savin-Williams, 1980b). In Chapter 7 an alterantive to the dominance structure for female groups is proposed.

The dominance structure among the early adolescent girls was not obvious to either group or nongroup members. Furthermore, the derived sociometric hierarchy was not highly correlated with the behavioral dominance hierarchy. The girls were less likely than boys to accurately perceive their self-rank, and more likely to underrank themselves. Dominance does not appear to have been a highly desirable or discernible trait to them.

The pattern for the adolescent boys was opposite on most accounts. Boys from 10 to 17 years of age were likely to accurately perceive their rank, immediately and years later. Relative status was clearly apparent to both group and nongroup members, both in the early adolescent data and the all-camp data. Hierarchies and groups became more stable over time; the frequency rate decreased during the camp sessions. The boys wanted to be considered dominant (overranking of self) and begged the counselors to tell them where everyone else rated them on dominance. Considering the all-camp data, 43% of the boys overranked themselves while only 11% underrated their group status.

Douvan (1960) has pointed out that the critical integrating variable for the adolescent girl is developing socioemotional and interpersonal sensitivity. Male adjustment is more dependent on achievement strivings, interdependence, energetic activity, competition, self-confidence, and assertion. Douvan attributes these differences to psychosocial ego development; others (Freedman, 1974; Hutt, 1972) ascribe a biological base as well. Delaying the consideration of "why" sex differences exist, the position taken here is that this task distinction between the sexes accounts for the variation in the female and male adolescents' group geist, behavioral patterns, and group structure.

Theoretical Issues

An examination of the daily schedule reveals that on the average the youth had slightly over three hours per day of "free time," when no all-camp or cabin group activity was planned. Boys spent this time engaged in sports such as basketball or tennis, usually with fellow cabinmates, or in asocial activities such as reading comic books or sleeping. On the other hand, it was uncommon for girls to spend this time with their cabin group or in organized and competitive activities; rather, they preferred to associate with sisters, cousins, home-town friends, extra-cabin friends, or a close cabin buddy in pairs or cliques, walking and talking. Thus, when involved with others, boys were in situations with a prefabricated organization, rules, and dominance structure; girls, with premiums placed on promoting interpersonal relationships, skills, and sensitivities. Perhaps the instability and low cohesiveness of the female groups can be attributed to a poor adaptation to the large camp setting and contrived cabin groups imposed on them by the camp adminstration. Given other context characteristics the adolescent girls may have prospered as a group. Perhaps it is not coincidental that the camp settings that were the most calm (low frequency of dominance interactions) were those that best predicted relative status.

This greater female concern with socioemotional issues is further substantiated by their resistance to completing the study's sociometrics. How much they liked cabinmates, who they thought were the leaders, and who they respected and why were "private" matters not to be publically divulged. The boys usually considered the sociometrics to be "fun things to do," requesting that the results be reported to the group as a whole (denied).

When asked to reach a group consensus on ideal leader traits, there were striking sex differences that conform to the diversity discussed above. Both sexes idealized honest, self-confident, and helpful leaders, but in other attributes they diverged along the instrumental-expressive dimension. Unique to male groups and largely instrumental were the traits: determined and tries hard at what he does, considerate in tolerating underlings, organizes activities, and knows what to do and makes the right decisions. The female groups emphasized expressive attributes: relates to my problems, friendly, outgoing, patient, considerate in respecting the needs and feelings of others, fun to be with, makes good judgments, and tries new things. When asked to characterize ideal friends there were few notable sex differences; the combined picture is strikingly similar to the girls' portrayal of an ideal leader: honest, trustworthy, fun, understanding, cooperative, kind, respectful (of you), sensible, and mature.[8] Thus, although both sexes perceived friendship in terms of socioemotional qualities, boys idealized an instrumental leader, but girls modeled an expressive leader who has the same attributes as a best friend.

Placing these sex differences in interpersonal encounters in the context of theoretical explanation can take several forms. Social conditioning theories are probably the most prevalent. For example, Hoffman (1979) notes that during early childhood both sexes are socialized for the expressive role, but that with increasing age boys are socialized into the

---

[8] These characteristics in turn are similar to a 1985 national poll conducted by Who's Who Among American High School Students. The top four responses to the question of what you look for in a friend were: reliability (86%), honesty (83%), sensitivity (75%), and sense of humor (75%).

emotion-inhibited, "instrumental character" necessary for occupational achievement. Pressures to conform to cultural stereotypes increase during adolescence because the peer group (Hartup, 1983), media (Katz, 1979), and parents (Kandel & Lesser, 1972) strongly portray the sexes in their traditional roles. It is not surprising, therefore, that adolescents engage in rigid sex-typing behavior (Urberg & Labouvie-Vief, 1976). The observed sex differences in dominance behavior and in verbal support and physical assistance may thus reflect the adolescent's response to the cultural expectation that girls express comfort or empathy and that boys react in a non-emotional, instrumental manner.

The ethologically-based male bonding theory of Tiger (1969) and the female contingency hypothesis of Angrist (1969) give a different theoretical account for the sex differences noted above. In primate groups Callan (1970) has noted that dominance relations among females tend to be relatively unorganized and unstructured when compared with inter-male behavior.

I should like to suggest, roughly, that one structural feature common to a good deal of human and animal social life is that the males are the conspicuous participators, the upholders of the contours and corners of the social map, and that the position of the female is characteristically more subtle or even equivocal with respect to this map. (p. 144)

Females may not be regularly engaged in dominance interactions among each other or with males, but they are the "keepers-in-being" of the system as a system by concerning themselves with the interpersonal aspects of group life.

The greater male proclivity for formulating and maintaining hierarchical and cohesive same-sex groups is empirically congruent with Tiger's (1969) speculations on group bonding and evolutionary theory. He proposes that male-male bonding is a positive valence or attraction, serving group defense, food-gathering, and social order maintenance purposes that are a direct consequence of pre-hominid ecological adaptation:

The two critical adaptations were the development of patterns of hunting large animals which may have involved tools and, more significantly, a propensity to form co-operative bonds which (as I will later argue) would have to be all-male. (p. 35)

Male-female physical and behavioral differences oriented the male toward participation in the hunting rather than the gathering (female) manner of exploiting the environment. Symons (1979) argues that the basic difference in a male and a female "human nature" is the result of the long evolutionary history of this hunting-gathering phase of our existence. Under hormonal influences the brain became masculinized or feminized resulting in dimorphism between the sexes in behavior.

Because of this orientation, adolescent males are more likely to adapt to mega-structural situations, such as camp, by forming linear organizations with clearly recognized status and authority structures (McGuinness, 1984). On the other hand, according to Angrist (1969), females are oriented toward a contingency sex role development. Rather than simply fitting into a highly organized and rule enforced structure, females negotiate interpersonal relationships in face-to-face interactions. Status may exist within a kinship system, but it is usually nonlinear. A linear system is dysfunctional, and was dysfunctional at Girls Camp at Wancaooah, because it negates the informal, socioemotional aspects of interpersonal relationships for cohesive and compatible female adolescent groups. The cohesive dyarchy form described in Chapter 7 allows for these unique female characteristics.

A recent restatement of these issues is Gilligan's (1982) book on moral development. Gilligan proposes that separation and individuation are central issues to a male's sense of identity. To be a male, boys must separate from the mother, are threatened by intimacy, and play games and sports in which they learn the importance of independence, organization, competition, fairness, and rules. Attachments and relationships are central to the adolescent girl. She is threatened by separation and individuation because they imply a rejection of what she is. She is concerned with caring, tolerance, responsibility, and cooperation; if she wins, then someone else must lose—which is not worth the cost (Sassen, 1980).

Gilligan (1982) notes that the vast majority of theoretical speculation as to the developmental tasks of adolescence implicitly assume a male perspective. Good adolescent development, according to Erikson (1959) entails separation, individuation, and a personalized ego identity. Thus, the adolescent girl is viewed as deficient and hence "less developed."

If the speculations of Angrist, Callan, Tiger, and Gilligan—which combine biological and social causations—are correct, then it would appear that in male peer groups positional status and structure are most important—a dominance hierarchy would service the needs of males—and among females, small intimate groups or dyads where connectedness and personalized interpersonal interactions reduce ambiguity. A cohesive dyarchy with shared responsibilities would best service the needs of females. In the context of a camp mega-structure, boys will feel more at home than will girls. Perhaps the difficult group experiences of the early adolescent girls in the current study reflect this difficulty. But at a less vulnerable age, older adolescent girls may adapt with their own version of a group structure. And it is to this that I now turn.

7
Age as a Factor in Dominance and Social Behavior

Chapter 6 discussed sex differences in the expression of dominance behaviors and the formation of a group structure; there are also age variations in these matters and in more generic social interactions. This chapter addresses these issues by reporting on data from groups of middle to late adolescents at summer camp and of early to middle adolescents engaged in school volleyball games.

Issues of Age

The existence of dominance and submission behaviors and a group dominance hierarchy are frequent assumptions and findings in a number of animal species, including fowl, nonhuman primates, and children. Beyond middle childhood, however, the view of non-ethologists Collins and Raven (1969) appears more prevalent: Whereas among groups of animals and human children a simple rank ordering based on power is characteristic, by adolescence the processes of socialization and cognitive development enhance the evolution of social systems—for example, authority, leadership, friendship, coalitions—with a complexity far more sophisticated than a dominance hierarchy. On the other hand, several ethologists cited in Chapter 2 proposed that although behaviors expressive of dominance will change with age, the basic social structure should be recognizably similar (Bernstein, 1981; Seyfarth, 1981; Smuts, 1981).

The present research casts doubt on the upper age restriction claims for a "simple" dominance hierarchy as descriptive of group structure, at least for male adolescents. This is not to imply, however, that behavior expressive of power and authority or that the physical, behavioral, and social predictors of status do not change with increasing age. Unfortunately, such age trends are difficult to assess given the dearth of naturalistic observation studies on dominance and submission among children and adolescents.

Four studies are described in this chapter that addresses this short-coming. The first has already been alluded to in Chapter 3: the two groups of male CITs at Camp Wancaooah. Another was designed by Roberta Paikoff (RP) with a group of adolescent girls at a Jewish camp. Age differences are more directly assessed in the final two studies that recorded behavioral interactions in different age groups of adolescents during school volleyball games.

Male Counselors-In-Training

The participants, two groups of 14-17 year old males at Camp Wan-caooah, and research design have been previously described in Chapter 3. The results of that investigation are now presented and discussed.

Group Structure: Observations

In both groups cabin members were rank-ordered on each of the eight indices of dominance behavior, placing first the boy who significantly dominated the greatest number of cabinmates in dyadic interactions; second, the boy who dominated the next highest number; and so forth, to the last-ranked boy, who dominated no one. In both groups these eight indice rank orders were significantly the same;[1] thus they were summed, resulting in the behavioral dominance hierarchy.

The dyadic matrices with the number and percentage of times that each adolescent boy dominated all other cabinmates is presented in Appendix B. Of the 25 dyads in the two groups, 20 (80%) were significant in directionality. The exceptions involved near-ranked boys in Group 9. Ties in the number of cabinmates significantly dominated were settled by giving higher placement to the boy who had the higher percentage.

In both groups the behavioral dominance hierarchy remained relatively unchanged over time and across behavior settings. Examining the data in 10-day periods, corresponding to temporal thirds of the camp session, the boys ranked significantly the same.[2] Regardless of whether data were collected during meals, discussions, or free time, group members ranked significantly the same.[3] The lowest percentage of hierarchical reversals, when a Y dominated an X, occurred during mealtimes (24% of all such behavior) and the highest, during free time (27%).

---

[1] Ws = .62 and .96, $p < .01$.
[2] Ws = .91 and .96, $p < .01$.
[3] Ws = .95 and .92, $p < .01$.

TABLE 7.1. Rates of Dominance Behaviors in Groups 9 and 10.

	Percent of total		Reversal rate	
	Group 9	Group 10	Group 9	Group 10
Ridicule	29%	33%	23%	17%
Verbal control	20%	18%	41%	29%
Recognition	20%	14%	26%	26%
Directive	14%	14%	24%	12%
Counter dominance	9%	9%	49%	23%
Physical assertiveness	4%	7%	59%	16%
Displacement	2%	3%	36%	25%
Threat	2%	2%	40%	25%

Group Structure: Sociometrics

A sociometric rank ordering of dominance was obtained by averaging the last week placements made by the youths, placing first the individual with the lowest numerical average; second, the next lowest average; and so forth. In both groups cabinmates significantly agreed among themselves on relative dominance ranking.[4] The composite group structure was significantly similar to the behavioral dominance hierarchy in both groups.[5]

Characteristics of the Behavioral Dominance Hierarchy

The most frequently observed indice of dominance was verbal ridicule; threats and displacements each contributed less than 3% of the total. Dominance behavior was least likely to occur during mealtimes (14.11 instances per observation hour), and most likely during cabin discussions (21.57 per hour).

Stability, as measured by the hierarchical reversal rate, remained essentially the same (Group 9) or slightly decreased (Group 10) from the first to the last third of camp. The two cabins, however, displayed discrepant temporal patterns. Even though the per hour frequency of dominance behavior increased during the three time periods of the camp session (from 18.35 to 25.68 to 33.53) in Group 9, the percentage of the total behavior that was overt decreased (from 59% to 67% to 55%, giving a 60% total). The pattern in Group 10 was the opposite: Over time the frequency of dominance behavior decreased (from 15.85 to 18.94 to 14.24), but the overtness level increased (from 59% to 69% to 68%, giving a 66%

---

[4] Xr^2s = 20.95 and 15.52, $p < .001$.
[5] Correlations were 1.00 and 0.70; combined $X^2 = 18.06, p < .01$.

TABLE 7.2. Correlation of Factors with the Behavioral Dominance Hierarchy

Factor	Group 9 r	Group 10 r	Combined χ^2	Significance p
Sociometric dominance	1.00	0.70	18.06	.01
Creativity	0.83	0.87	13.00	.02
Cabin leadership	0.49	0.97	12.64	.02
Spirit	0.83	0.70	11.25	.03
Intelligence	0.92	0.10	10.68	.04
Frequency of interactions	0.89	0.40	10.52	.04
Camp experience	0.64	0.82	10.44	.04
Peer friendship	0.49	0.90	9.87	.05
Crafts skill	0.54	0.82	9.42	.05
Overtness level	−0.49	−0.60	0.79	.05
Hiking position	0.49	0.80	8.75	ns
Chronological age	0.71	0.30	7.48	ns
Athletic ability	0.55	0.50	6.87	ns
Pubertal maturation	0.31	0.50	5.49	ns
Outcamping ability	0.43	0.07	4.55	ns
Socioeconomic status	0.31	−0.30	3.44	ns
Physical size	−0.09	0.20	3.12	ns
Bed position	−0.20	−0.90	1.01	ns

total). The difference in frequency is illustrated by the fact that in Group 9, 73% of the pairs increased their dyadic interactions from the first to the last third of camp while in Group 10, 80% of the pairs decreased their frequency.[6]

Predictors of the Behavioral Dominance Hierarchy

On all nine sociometric exercises group members significantly agreed among themselves on relative rank.[7] Of these, creativity, cabin leadership, spirit, intelligence, peer friendship, and crafts skill were significantly correlated with the behavioral dominance hierarchy (Table 7.2).

Relative differences in pubertal maturation, physical size, chronological age, socioeconomic status, bed position, and hiking position were not significantly related to the behavioral dominance hierarchy. Camp experience indicated higher rank and dominant boys expressed their dominance more frequently and less overtly than lower ranking group members.

On the dominance sociometric 18% of the boys overranked themselves in relation to their group standing, 27% underranked themselves, and 55% were accurate in self-placement. Considering all sociometrics the fifth-,

---

[6]$X^2 = 6.84, p < .01.$
[7]Xr^2s ranged from 10.56 to 21.42, $p < .01.$

sixth-, and second-ranked boys were most likely to overrank themselves (65%, 50%, and 43%, respectively).

A Group of Late Adolescent Females[8]

Method

The study was conducted at a coeducational summer camp in the eastern United States. The four-week camp gives a basic Jewish and Zionist education. Daily activities consisted of religious services, educational programs, singing, dancing, and dramatics in the mornings; optional sports and free time in the afternoon; and various cultural and educational programs in the evening. There were also many special program days at camp: weekly Sabbath, Parents' Day, a two-day hike, and a Holocaust Memorial Day.

Eight female adolescents (six 17-year-olds and two 16-year-olds) from suburban, middle and upper-middle class Jewish backgrounds were participants in this study. All eight individuals lived in one cabin, with RP as their counselor; they were assigned by age to this cabin group by the camp adminstration. None of the youth had previously been to this particular summer camp. The cabin that the participants lived in was connected to another cabin of females, and across from a cabin of males. These three groups participated in most activities together, including eating meals with each other.

The same eight indices of dominance behaviors were used here as measures of one individual's assertion over another. Slight modifications were made on the specifics of the behavior indices, combining certain subcategories and adding others.

Each girl rated herself and all bunkmates on the following traits, using a scale of 1 (low) to 5 (high):

1. Knowledge: "How well do you know _____?"
2. Empathy: "How empathic is she?"
3. Friendship: "How good a friend of yours is she?"
4. Dominance: "How much influence does she have in bunk decisions?"
5. Creativity: "How often does she volunteer new and original ideas?"
6. Intelligence: "How intelligent is she?"

---

[8] This research formed the basis for Roberta Paikoff's Senior Honors Thesis for the Department of Human Development and Family Studies at Cornell University, October, 1982. The study is further described in Paikoff and Savin-Williams (1983).

7. Popularity: "How popular is she in bunk, in unit, with girls outside unit, with boys outside unit?"
8. Attractiveness: "How physically attractive is she?"
9. Spirit: "How much fun is she to be with?"
10. Leadership: "How much of a leader is she?"
11. Self-consistency: "Do her actions correspond with what she says is the correct way to behave?"
12. Angry/Hurt: "When she is constructively criticized by others, does she get angry? hurt?"
13. Athletic ability: "How good is she at sports?"

All completed the Coopersmith Self-Esteem Inventory (SEI), a widely used self-report instrument of global self-esteem: "A personal judgment of worthiness that is expressed in the attitude the individual holds toward himself" (Coopersmith, 1967; p. 5). There are 54 statements (e.g. "I often wish I were someone else.") that require one of two responses: "like me" or "unlike me." The SEI is a self-report measure with acceptable test-retest reliability (Taylor & Reitz, 1968), and good convergent, discrim-inant, and predictive validity (Robinson & Shaver, 1973).

The Schwartz Ascription of Responsibility Scale (1968) was also given to the girls. The Schwartz is a self-report instrument with a list of statements with responses on a continuum of 1 to 4, where 1 is "strongly agree" and 4 is "strongly disagree." Although some of the statements on the Schwartz are "I feel" statements, there are also abstract statements that allow the individual to agree or disagree with a philosophy as opposed to reporting behavior (e.g. "Professional obligations can never justify neglecting the welfare of others").

Observations of dominance behavior were recorded five days per week by RP for approximately 100 minutes per day (four week total = 25.2 hours). Each girl was observed individually during a 10-minute time span and all dominance interactions that she had with cabin members, regardless of directionality, were noted discretely. RP carried a clipboard to each meal and activity, habituating the girls to its presence. A letter was always being written on the top sheet of the clipboard with recorded observations several pages beneath it to insure privacy.

The order of girls observed was randomly arranged, but with the imposed stipulation that each girl was observed at least two but not more than three times every other day, for an equal amount of time over the three settings (bunk, mealtimes, and activities). A usual day consisted of 20 to 30 minutes of in-bunk (waking, rest, and nighttime periods) observations, 30 minutes of mealtime observations, and 30 to 60 minutes of observations in activities with other campers. The amount of time of individual observation for the camp session ranged from 180 to 204 minutes per girl, averaging 189.

Observer reliability was assessed prior to the beginning of the camp session between RP and SW at a local school and at a youth movement conference with a population similar to that of the camp where the current study took place. Four behaviors occurred frequently enough to determine item reliability (recognition, counter dominance, verbal control, and verbal directive). These four behaviors comprised 85% of all observations during this study. The overall reliability score was .78, with separate behavior scores ranging from .64 for directives to .88 for recognition and counter dominance.

The paper-and-pencil exercises were completed during an activities hour by the adolescents. Peer-rating sheets were given to each girl at this time during the first and fourth weeks of camp. The Schwartz was completed during the second week and the SEI, during the third week. All youth were given the option of whether or not to participate in the exercises (all chose to, with the exception of one individual who did not finish the fourth week rating sheet). General feedback was provided to each girl in the form of a camper evaluation by RP at the conclusion of camp.

Frequency

The frequency of dominance interactions recorded during the four-week camp session was 13.13 behaviors per hour. The frequency rate increased

TABLE 7.3. Frequency and Reversal Rates for Selected Dominance Behaviors for all Settings and Times

	Frequency (per hour)		Reversal rate (%)
Behavior			
Recognition	5.37	40%	33
First two weeks	3.24		35
Second two weeks	1.96		25
Counter dominance	2.42	18%	29
Verbal control	2.17	17%	26
Verbal ridicule	1.57	12%	27
Total overt behaviors	4.69		
First two weeks	4.06		
Second two weeks	5.60		
Setting			
Bunk	7.97		32
Meals	3.17		29
Activities	2.00		29
Time			
First two weeks	12.72		34
Second two weeks	13.70		21
Total	13.13		28

over time: 12.72 behaviors per hour for the first two weeks and 13.70 for the second two weeks. Recognition behaviors were the most frequently observed (40% of total behaviors, see Table 7.3). Physical contact, displacement, and threat behaviors were least frequent; when combined they constituted 4% of the total behaviors observed.

Group Structure

Unidirectional dominance relationships for the group were determined by assigning each girl an overall dominance score based on the following criteria: Two points were given for each statistically significant uni-directional dominance relationship and one point for every dominance trend. After these points were totaled for each girl, two points were subtracted from that score for each statistically submissive relationship and one point for each submissive trend.

In relationships that were within one point of each other, the pertinent dyad was examined to see if one girl was dominant over the other (see Appendix B). In the case of the top two behaviorally ranked girls, differences were not significant, thus, the two were regarded as equally effective in behavioral dominance interactions. Of the 56 dyads in the cabin, 43% were unidirectional.

Stability of Dominance Relationships

Over time the girls in the bunk ranked in the same order. The reversal rate, the percentage of the total number of dominance behaviors occurring in a group that transgresses the structure, for the four weeks of observations was 28%. Some evidence suggests that the bunk structure became more stable over time: The reversal rate for the first two weeks of camp was 34% and for the second two weeks, 21%. Dominance relationships were most stable during activities and least stable in the bunk.

Only four behaviors occurred frequently enough to assess their stability: recognition, counter dominance, verbal control, and ridicule. Of the four, verbal control was the most stable (reversal rate, 26%), and recognition was the least stable (33%). Recognition behaviors, however, became more stable during the course of camp, the reversal rate declining to 25% during the second two weeks.

Overtness

During the four-week camp session, 38% of the dominance behavior was overt and involved open recognition, either physical or verbal, of a dominance relationship. The overtness of the girls' behavior increased over time, from 32% in the first two weeks to 45% during the second half of camp. When examined on an individual level, there were differences in successful utilization of overt/covert dominance behaviors. The percentage of successful overt behaviors for each girl follows: Alice 52%, Betty, 21%, Gretchen, 38%, Denise 49%, Ellen 25%, Zoe 20%, Theresa 17%, and Ina 24%.

Paper-and-Pencil Exercises

Participants were ranked from highest to lowest on each trait. A Spearman rank order correlation (Siegel, 1956) was computed for all traits, comparing the first- and fourth-week rankings. No significant differences were found between the two on any measure; thus, all data analyses used the fourth-week ratings.

The peer rating sheets were also analyzed by isolating the dominance ratings each individual gave to all cabin members. Based on these numerical ratings, the girls were rank ordered to determine the power structure of the cabin, as perceived by each girl. All possible rank order comparisons were made between the seven girls. Of the 28 comparisons 26 were significant at the .05 level with correlations between .68 and .97. The two pairs that did not reach significance were at the .10 level, with correlations of .52 and .64.

Each of the peer-rated traits was compared with behavioral dominance. Participants were ranked on the Schwartz and SEI measures and on the overtness of their behavior. In addition, participants were ranked on how much they either over- or underrated themselves in comparison to the mean group score they received on a particular trait.

The following characteristics were significantly correlated with behavioral dominance: sociometric dominance (.96), well-known (.95), friendship (.92), leadership (.90), athletic ability (.88), spirit, (.87), self-esteem (.83), empathy (.80), under- to overratings (.76), and self-consistency (.67). The following variables did not significantly correlate with behavioral dominance: physical attractiveness (.59), creativity (.56), intelligence (.54), popularity with girls (.54), overtness (.49) angry/hurt (.40), popularity with boys (.24), and the Schwartz (.08).

A best friend was most likely to be an individual next to one in dominance rank (expected by chance: 25%; observed: 63%). That is, closely ranked adolescent girls tended to be best friends.

Male Volleyball Games[9]

Ethologists search for normative environments in which to observe their animal. One context in which human adolescents choose to spend a

---

[9]For a more complete report of this study see Savin-Williams, 1982.

considerable portion of their time is in active leisure (Csikszentmihalyi & Larson, 1984). They must also, however, spend a large part of their day in school. Combining these two, physical education classes is an obvious setting for observing adolescent behavior. Two variables, one person-centered (age) and one context-based (winning, losing, tying), were investigated by observing adolescent behavior during physical education classes. Of interest was whether male adolescents differed in the amount and type of social interactions of a more generalized nature than dominance behaviors as a function of their age and of game conditions.

Setting and Participants

Four 8th grade and four 10th grade, all-male physical education volley-ball teams were observed during age-based round-robin tournament play. The 52 boys, each on one of the eight teams, were students at a midwestern university laboratory school for professorial and staff children. The sample is homogeneous in socioeconomic status but diverse in ethnicity (80% Caucasian, 10% Black, and 10% Hispanic).

Twenty-four games, lasting 7-14 minutes each, were observed by two individuals trained in observational data collecting techniques.[10] An equal amount of time was spent watching 8th and 10th grade games. All observations were made from a balcony overlooking the playing floor of the gymnasium. The height of the balcony afforded a good view of the game without being obtrusive, although sufficiently close so that all verbal utterances by the participants were audible.

Procedures

Beginning with the first serve of the game, the two observers, one for each team, recorded all verbal and physical behavior directed at another team member or to the team as a whole.[11] In order to limit the large amount of social interactions occurring, all exchanges between teams or with the referee were excluded. We focused just on intra-team behavior inter-

---

[10] I thank co-observer Janet Bare Ashear for her data collection during the volleyball games and for her critical insights. Mr. Zarvis, the school's physical education director, was kind enough to let us observe his classes. He was, at all times, cooperative and encouraging. Our study participants, unbeknown to them, only had to be themselves.

[11]Reliability was assessed midway through the investigation when the two observers made simultaneous recordings of the same team for two games (16 minutes). The reliability was 72% agreement in the first game and 77% agreement in the second game.

actions, which were narrated into a tape recorder as they occurred, along with the score that time elapsed. The observation period ended with the game-winning, usually the 15th, point.

A coding scheme employing event-sampling and placement of behavior into categories (Wright, 1960) was used. The initiated behavior and the response were recorded. Six categories of initiated behavior were distinguished, modeled from Gellert (1961):

a) Encouragement to the group as a whole: "We've got to work together if we want to win!"
b) Discouragement to the group as a whole, usually accompanied with an obscenity: "Damn! We'll never win this one!"
c) Positive instruction or advice to another: "Mickey, hit the ball with two hands."
d) Negative criticism, teasing, or boasting to another: "Mark, you idiot! You can't hit nothin'!"
e) Neutral statements or questions: "What's the score?"
f) Physical contact, given in a neutral (push into place), positive (giving "skin"), or negative (hitting) manner.

The responses were one of three varieties:

a) Non-compliance, rejection, or counter dominance: "Mind your own damn business!"
b) Submission or compliance to the instructions, criticisms, or physical contact of another: "Sure, I'll try to use both hands next time."
c) Neutral response with no acknowledgement of the initiated behavior.

For all age $\times$ game conditions possibilities, per-minute frequencies of initiated and response events were calculated. Significance for independence was tested by using the chi-square goodness-of-fit statistic in a row-by-column contingency table format.

Permission for the study was obtained through the school's physical education director. The university laboratory school students are frequent participants in research projects. Thus, the volleyball players appeared quite undisturbed by the presence of the balcony observers. Their involvement in the tournament games was usually captivating, diverting their attention from the observers.

Frequency of Behaviors

During the 226 minutes of observations, 915 instances of intra-team social interactions were recorded, yielding a 4.05 per-minute frequency rate. Of the six categories of initiated behavior, encouragement to the group (38%) and neutral statements (24%) were the most frequently observed (Table 7.4). Discouragement to the group (6%) rarely occurred.

TABLE 7.4. Number and Percentage of Initiated and Response Behaviors Occurring for Each Age and Game Condition Variable

| | Age | | | | | | Game condition | | | | | |
| | Total | | 8th | | 10th | | Win | | Loss | | Tie | |
Initiated	N	%	N	%	N	%	N	%	N	%	N	%
Encouragement	350	38	174	35	176	42	172	46	132	34	46	31
Discouragement	58	6	30	6	28	7	13	3	33	9	12	9
Positive Instructions	77	9	37	8	40	9	32	9	31	8	14	9
Negative Criticisms	132	15	91	18	41	10	30	8	79	20	23	16
Neutral Statements	222	24	105	21	117	28	92	24	91	23	39	26
Physical Contact	76	8	57	12	29	4	39	10	23	6	14	9
	915	100%	494	100%	421	100%	378	100%	389	100%	148	100%
Responses	N	%	N	%	N	%	N	%	N	%	N	%
Non-Compliance	43	5	33	7	10	2	13	3	27	7	3	2
Submission	240	26	123	25	117	28	86	23	103	26	51	34
Neutral	632	69	338	68	294	70	279	74	259	67	94	64
	915	100%	494	100%	421	100%	378	100%	389	100%	148	100%
Per Hour Frequency of Behavior	4.03		4.37		3.73		3.74		3.93		5.69	

The most frequent response was neutral (69%) with few non-compliance responses (5%).

The per-hour frequency rate was higher among 8th than 10th grade youths and during tied games rather than those being won or lost (Table 7.4). Social interactions most frequently occurred when 8th grade games were tied and least likely to occur when 10th graders were winning their games.

Age Effects

The early and middle adolescents significantly differed in the kinds of behavior that they initiated and in their responses when playing same-age volleyball games.[12] Eighth-graders were three times more likely than 10th grade students to make physical contact in the form of "giving skin," punching, and patting on the back. They were also far more critical of teammates, and frequently responded to requests or instructions with non-compliant behavior. Tenth-graders were more likely to initiate encouragements and neutral statements.

Game Conditions Effects

Game conditions had a significant effect on behaviors initiated and on the responses of the participants.[13] Winning and losing game situations were mirror images of each other in the kinds of behavior that they evoked from the participants. When winning, players were likely to encourage teammates, to make physical contact, and to seldom discourage or criticize others. Losing evoked a high level of discouragement, criticism, non-compliance, and a low level of encouragement and physical contact. Tied games elicited little encouragement and non-compliance and a high level of submission.

Age and Game Condition Interaction Effects

There was a significant age by game condition effect.[14] In particular, the high level of social interactions during 8th grade tied games and during 10th grade games that were being lost accounted for the majority of the chi-square statistic.

---

[12]X^2 (5) = 22.88, $p < .001$; X^2 (2) = 10.24, $p < .01$.
[13]X^2 (10) = 42.41, $p < .001$; X^2 (4) = 15.83, $p < .01$)
[14]X^2 (2) = 9.04, $p < .02$.

Female Volleyball Games[15]

The adolescent girl interacting with other adolescent girls has been, and continues to be, largely ignored by developmental psychologists and ethologists (Savin-Williams, 1980b). When the interaction occurs in a sports context, the silence is intense: There are few existing studies of adolescent female sports behavior. Yet, play and games are considered to be important building blocks in the socialization process of becoming human (Matza, 1964; Mead, 1934; Roberts & Sutton-Smith, 1962). Sports, as one example of play and games, has historically been limited to males; females have been discouraged, prohibited, and underrepresented because participation in sports is incompatible with commonly accepted female sex-role stereotype (Johnson & Cofer, 1974; Loy, McPherson & Kenyon, 1978). The traditional cultural prescription for the feminine sex role embraces passivity, weakness, and dependency and excludes competitiveness, aggression, and independence (Snyder & Kivlin, 1977). Femininity has been considered throughout our history to be a physically inactive state; those who dare to participate are less than women, and are certainly unfeminine (Elkins, 1978; Felshin, 1973).

As a child if a girl expresses interest in sports she is generally permitted by parents to participate (Loy et al., 1978). If, however, this interest continues into adolescence she faces negative cultural sanctions (Cheska, 1970).

Females are permitted to be "tomboys" in childhood; when they enter adolescence, women may be discouraged from developing their bodies for strength or athletic prowess. "Slimnastics" takes the place of the athletic skills building during this period (Romer, 1981; p. 66). The adolescent girl's decrease in activity level is more of a cultural phenomenon than a biological necessity; our society tells a girl to become a "young lady" and this implies a non-athletic mode (Aivers, Barnett, & Baruch, 1979).

Existing research indicates that the public in general and female athletes in particular, perceive that female participation in sports carries with it a powerful stigma (Snyder & Kilvin, 1977; Snyder & Spreitzer, 1973). One social stigma that appears to be especially threatening to the adolescent girl actively involved in the sports is the label of lesbian (Elkins, 1978). Or, she may feel that she is less attractive to boys if she engages in serious sports behavior; not only is she less feminine, but she may also be perceived as a threat to the masculinity concerns of the

---

[15]For a more complete report of this study see Savin-Williams, Bolger, & Spinola, 1986. My appreciation is extended to Geraldine Downey for her comments on this study; to the girls, the physical education teachers, the two school principles, and the board of education in each town for their cooperation; and to Susan Spinola who collected the data.

adolescent male. Thus, the preadolescent "tomboy" becomes the adolescent lesbian or the promless girl in the eyes of many (Hicks, 1979).

Unfortunately, we have little information on the athletic behavior of girls who are early or middle adolescents, especially when it involves interpersonal behavior in naturalistic contexts (Savin-Williams, 1980b). The primary purpose in the present investigation is to examine age-related changes in sports behavior for groups of girls. In contrast to the findings for boys, the older adolescent girls should demonstrate *less involvement* in sports and adopt a *more feminine* and *less masculine* approach to athletic activities they cannot ignore. These age differences in social behavior, it is hypothesized, can be attributable in part to changes in internalized sex-role prescriptions.

Setting and Participants

The study was conducted in 6th, 8th, and 10th grade physical education volleyball classes in two public schools, an elementary school (K-8) and a high school (9-12). The schools are located in small, suburban towns along the New Jersey shore.

Twenty-one middle-class, Caucasian girls are included in the study, seven in each grade. In the 6th and 8th grade physical education classes 30 girls played in the volleyball games with 15 girls on each team. Every girl in the 6th and 8th grades drew a number from a hat; the seven who chose numbers one through seven were included in the study. The seven participants always played on the same team, whereas the rest of the girls dispersed themselves on the participants' teams or formed the opposition teams. In the 10th grade there were 14 girls who participated in the volleyball games. The seven randomly selected youth were always on the same team playing against the other seven.

Observation Measures and Procedures

The youth were observed from the sidelines of a volleyball court. Recorded into a tape recorder were all observations of social behavior. To facilitate the recording of data and to preserve anonymity, the seven adolescent girls in each grade wore numbered vests.

Initially, 17 behavioral categories were delineated, based on a natural grouping of behavior and on previous observation studies (Gellert, 1961, Savin-Williams, 1980b). For data analysis purposes the 17 were coded according to the six categories used by the companion study of adolescent males. Three varieties, however, rarely occurred: discouragement to the group as a whole, neutral statements or questions, and physical contact. The following five categories were used in this study, based on the study of adolescent males (the first three) and on a categorization of behavior that was not observed among the males (the last two).[16]

1. *Encouragement to the group.* Examples include cheering, encouraging ("Let's work together!"), and sympathizing ("That's allright, we'll get that point back!") verbal behaviors, and nonverbal behaviors such as clapping hands, jumping up and down, and patting teammates on the back.
2. *Assisting a teammate.* Verbal—"Use both hands next time; it's easier"— and nonverbal—demonstrating an easy way to serve—forms are included.
3. *Negative expression.* Verbal name calling ("Jerk!"), criticism ("That was a lousy serve!"), sarcasm ("Real nice, for them"), physical contact (pricking another girl), and non-physical means (raising middle finger) are examples.
4. *Distracting behavior.* Verbal—"I just got a pair of jeans"—and nonverbal—fixing hair, picking fingernails, falling down on the floor for the fun of it—means are assessed.
5. *Avoidance behavior.* Examples include screaming in fright when the ball comes nearby, ducking away from the ball, or covering the head when the ball approaches.

Each grade was observed for three class periods so as to minimize a particular day's effects. The majority of the participants in each grade were observed for five minutes in each period for a total of 15 minutes; the five minute intervals were timed with a stop watch. Some of the girls, however, were only observed during one or two class periods (5 or 10 minutes total) because the class periods were too short to observe all seven girls for five minutes each. The one or two who were not observed during a class period were the first girls to be observed in the next class period.

The average total observation time per individual girl was 11.7, 13.6, and 12.1 minutes in the 6th, 8th, and 10th grades, respectively. The observation times ranged from 5 to 15 minutes among the 6th and 10th graders, and between 10 to 15 minutes among the 8th graders.

Bem Sex Role Inventory

The Bem Sex Role Inventory (BSRI) (Bem, 1981) assesses the extent that respondents have the typical characteristics of the socialized sex roles of American culture. The BSRI was chosen because previous studies have

---

[16] Interjudge reliability of observer ratings was assessed as follows: SS and another female observer made simultaneous recordings for each of the 21 girls during one time period. The overall interjudge observer reliability score was .73 with individual girls' totals ranging from .61 to .89.

indicated that individuals classified as sex-typed by the BSRI tend to be sex-typed in their behavior (Bem, Martyna & Watson, 1976) and motivated to select sex-typed activities (Bem & Lenney, 1976).

The BSRI identifies sex-typed participants on the basis of self-ratings of personal attributes. Each participant indicates on a scale from never or almost never true to always or almost always true how well each of the attributes describes her personality. These attributes reflect the Western cultural definition of masculinity (e.g., aggressive, assertive, athletic, competitive, independent) or of femininity (e.g., affectionate, cheerful, gentle, loyal, warm) or serve as neutral descriptions—neither masculine nor feminine attributes (e.g., helpful, reliable, sincere, tactful, friendly).

The BSRI was given to each of the 21 participants on the last day of observations. The majority of the girls had difficulty understanding several of the BSRI adjectives (e.g., self-reliant, yielding, theatrical, compassionate, assertive, analytical, flatterable, self-sufficient). These terms were explained with a common definition. After completing the BSRI, a masculine and a feminine score was derived for each respondent—the mean score of the masculine and feminine items, respectively.

Age Differences

Table 7.5 presents means and standard deviations for the five behavior categories for early and middle adolescents. For analytical purposes, the data for the 8th and 10th grade students were pooled because preliminary analyses indicated that these groups had essentially identical behavior profiles. In addition, the data were adjusted to equate the groups on length of observation time.

The hypothesis that the two age groups differ in terms of the five behaviors was tested.[17] As shown in Table 7.5 early (6th grade) and middle (8th and 10th grade) adolescents differed significantly on these measures.[18] Having established that the groups differ in this overall sense, the groups were then tested on each of the five behaviors considered individually.[19] Of the five behaviors, encouragement ($t = 4.9$) and distracting behavior ($t = -2.6$) differed between early and middle adolescent girls. Specifically, middle adolescents were less likely to give

---

[17]Hotellings T-squared, a multivariate generalization of the independent-groups t-test was used.

[18]$F(5, 15) = 5.40, p < .05$.

[19] The overall probability of a Type I error was fixed at .05 or less using the Bonferroni method of simultaneous hypothesis testing. The critical value of t for each test ($df = 19$) is 2.53, where each of our hypotheses is directional, that is, middle adolescents were expected to show less involvement in the game than early adolescents.

TABLE 7.5. Raw Means and Means Adjusted for Masculinity and Femininity

Numbers of Behaviors: Raw Means (SDs in parentheses)

	Encouragement	Assistance	Negativity	Distraction	Avoidance
Early adolescents	34.1	2.5	7.1	9.0	0.3
	(17.0)	(2.7)	(4.7)	(5.2)	(0.8)
Middle adolescents	9.7	1.5	6.4	24.0	3.7
	(6.1)	(1.5)	(8.2)	(14.7)	(4.5)
Between-group difference	24.4	1.0	0.7	−15.0	−3.4
Univariate t (df = 19)	4.9*	1.1	0.2	−2.6*	−1.9
Multivariate F(5,15) = 5.40*					
Early adolescents	34.8	2.6	8.0	11.0	1.0
	(3.9)	(0.8)	(2.8)	(4.6)	(1.3)
Middle adolescents	9.3	1.4	5.9	23.0	3.3
	(2.7)	(.5)	(2.0)	(3.2)	(0.9)
Between-group difference	25.4	1.1	2.1	−12.0	−2.3
Univariate t (df = 17)	5.3*	1.2	0.6	−2.1	−1.4
Multivariate F(5,13) = 4.74*					

*Overall Type I error rate set at .05

encouragement to their teammates and more likely to engage in distracting behavior.

The Sex-Role Hypothesis

A key hypothesis of the study was whether observed age differences in sport behaviors are attributable to changes in sex-role orientation. To test this hypothesis, it was ascertained whether, and to what extent, the age difference remained when measures of sex-role orientation were introduced as statistical controls.[20] When considered simultaneously, the behaviors were not significantly related to masculinity or femininity, nor did the age effect diminish substantially in their presence.[21]

The extent to which the age difference for each individual behavior remained in the presence of the sex-role covariates was used.[22] The groups differed on encouragement alone ($t = 5.3$).

As shown in Table 7.5 in the adjusted means, the between-group differences in encouragement increased slightly when group differences in masculinity and femininity were taken into account. In contrast, between-group differences in distracting behavior decreased from 15 units to 12 units in the presence of the sex-role measures, and, in consequence, became sufficiently small to accept the null hypothesis. Thus, there is evidence that the original age difference in this measure can be explained, in part, by group differences in sex-role orientation. Unfortunately, there is insufficient degrees of freedom in the present study to estimate regression coefficients for the sex-role variables while simultaneously maintaining a low probability of a Type I error.

Age Trends in Dominance Behavior

In most respects the data reported in the first two studies are similar to previous research on groups of children and early adolescents. Although the specific behaviors used to express one's dominance status differ depending on one's age (Abramovitch, 1980; Cairns, 1979; Weisfeld & Weisfeld, 1984), from the earliest age of social behavior through the end of childhood and the onset of biological maturation, when individuals are placed in same-age and same-sex groups dyadic power relationships develop that have meaning on a group level. The present data extended

---

[20] The model employed is a multivariate generalization of the analysis of covariance (MANCOVA).

[21] $F(5, 13) = 2.17$ (N.S.); $F(5, 13) = 2.64$ (N.S.); $F(5, 13) = 4.74, p < .05$.

[22] Univariate ANVOVA's were employed. The Bonferroni method was employed to maintain the overall level of Type I error at .05. The critical value of t for each of the five tests (one-tail) was 2.57.

the developmental time line past the onset of pubescence to the middle and late adolescent years. The male group structure, although far from a rigid peck order, is a dominance hierarchy that was readily perceived by group members and remained relatively unchanged over time and across behavior settings. Alterations were minor, consisting of near-ranked individuals exchanging positions. The female group structure, however, assumed a somewhat different form, a "cohesive dyarchy."

For both early and late adolescents the group structure was most stable during free time and athletic activities and least stable during discussions in the cabin group. The latter was also the setting with the highest frequency rate of dominance interactions; mealtimes again proved to be the most peaceful. For both sexes verbal ridicule remained the most common form of asserting status; physical and verbal threats and displacements were seldom used to subordinate others. There was a slight tendency for older adolescents to more frequently underrank self on the dominance sociometric, but most group members accurately perceived their group status rank.

Females

There is some indication, based on the group of the late adolescent females, that a different structure, termed a "cohesive dyarchy," is characteristic of dominance relations among adolescent girls. One way in which this structure differs from a dominance hierarchy is that individuals are ordered in a less linear arrangement. The horizontality of the cohesive dyarchy implies that more than one person can occupy a rank.

The best friend pairs so prevalent among early adolescent girls are still evident among the late adolescents; absent, however, are the constant changing of best friends and the backbiting, bickering, and cattiness. Best friend cliques were transformed among the late adolescents into a more cohesive, complex style of group functioning. For example, the two top ranked girls were equally effective in asserting dominance, but did so in different ways. This reflects the greater division of labor in accordance with female needs of expressivity; it acknowledges the equal importance of looking out for each others' feelings and of "getting the job done." In the sociological literature the concepts of instrumental and expressive leaders are employed to distinguish these two types of leaders (Parsons & Bales, 1955). An instrumental leader reduces the likelihood of group conflict due to lack of direction by giving structure to group activities; an expressive leader reduces the likelihood of conflict between individuals, and thus allows the group to function as a cohesive unit.

This dichotomy is helpful in understanding the behavioral differences between Alice and Betty in the late adolescent female group. Alice, as the instrumental leader, was successful in overt behaviors involving ridicule and control; Betty filled the expressive role, successful in subtle behaviors, involving others' recognition of her status and her own counter dominance. The girls approached Alice and Betty for different reasons. They were far more likely to ask Betty for advice on friendship, clothing, and hairstyle, and to approach Alice to ask her to do something with them (e.g., swimming, walking) or to seek approval of ideas for group activities. It is plausible that in male groups the instrumental leader is the alpha-ranked individual; if there is an expressive leader he is clearly subordinate in the dominance hierarchy, perhaps because emotionality is not a highly valued male characteristic, or he combines it with instrumentality to become the alpha boy.

Thus, the cohesion and stability that were absent in the early adolescent female peer groups were characteristic of the late adolescent female group. In early adolescence, ridicule was the most frequently exhibited behavior; in late adolescence, recognition was far more frequent than ridicule. Dominance was manifested by older girls through subtle means; sensitivity and tolerance, rather than mere politeness, were important group values. Perhaps once girls have defined who they are in late adolescence, they are less likely to turn on other girls and are more likely to engage in altruistic, helping behavior.

Pubertal maturation was not an important predictor of dominance in late adolescent girls, as it was in early adolescence. But, there was little variation in pubescence because all late adolescent girls except one were nearly fully developed. Pubertal timing—early, on time, and late—was not assessed. As with early adolescents, peer ratings of friendship and athletic ability significantly predicted which late adolescent girls would be most dominant. Although peer popularity with girls and with boys did not reach significance, the most dominant girls were well-known and were perceived as the leaders and those with the most spirit. These instrumental attributes co-exist in predicting high status with a more expressive characteristic, empathy. Unlike the findings of Weisfeld, Bloch, and Ivers (1984) with the same age girls, physical attractiveness did not predict dominance status; neither were the more cognitively oriented variables (intelligence and creativity) significant predictors of dominance. The most dominant girls had the highest self-esteem, but they did not ascribe to themselves a greater sense of responsibility—perhaps because the responsibility was more in abstract terms than in reference to the immediate context of group life.

These findings should be accepted only with great caution. Only one group of late adolescent girls was observed and they differed in significant ways (e.g., religion, camp setting, hometowns) from the early adolescents. Replication should extend this investigation to other groups of late adolescent females.

Males

There were also important age differences in characteristics and predictors of the male dominance hierarchy. Physical assertiveness was three times more likely to occur among early than late adolescent males. On the other hand, recognition of status behavior was three times more prevalent among late than early male adolescent dyads. In addition, late adolescent boys were considerably less overt when interacting than were early adolescent males (63% and 86% overt ratios, respectively). This pattern of recognizing the status of others, but not of being overt or physical when dominating others, is more similar to female than to male early adolescent behavior.

Unique to late adolescent groups were the characteristics that significantly predicted dominance rank. Unlike both male and female early adolescent groups, relative individual differences in pubertal maturation did not predict dominance status. Neither were other physically based variables such as chronological age, physical size, hiking position, and outcamping skill related to dominance rank. Rather, individual variations in mental traits, camp experience, and social skills were important correlates of dominance status. The youngest and oldest male cabins in the all-camp data reflect these findings. With age pubertal maturation becomes less important, dropping from a .60 to a .27 correlation, and peer popularity (.39 to .67) and intelligence (.07 to .31) became better predictors of dominance status.

Females and Males

During the early pubescent years physical traits were important in distinguishing relative rank. One explanation for this is the dramatic saliency of physical variability during this time. For example, among the groups of 12 to 13 year old boys, pubertal maturation stage (Tanner, 1962) ranged from 1 to 4; among the 14 to 17 year old boys the stages were either 4 or 5. Relative differences in height and weight were just as marked; from 58-71 inches and 81-140 pounds among the early adolescents, but from 66-73 inches and 121-165 pounds among the late adolescents. When physical features become more equalized at the conclusion of pubescence, other variables such as friendship, cabin spirit, leadership, and intelligence[23] are emphasized, demarcating individual variation and, consequently, importance in regard to group dominance status. The drop in the use of pushing and shoving and of overt categories among late

---

[23]Although the sexes differ on significance level, the correlation for intelligence is nearly identical: .51 for males and .54 for females. Similarly, sex differences in the predictive correlation of creativity and athletic ability are not great, especially given the small sample size.

adolescents underscores this deemphasis of physical modes of asserting dominance position, also found by others (e.g., Cairns, 1979). Girls develop this deemphasized physical pattern earlier, perhaps because of their earlier physical maturation or their earlier learning of the importance of social and mental characteristics, or to both.

Although athletic ability is a good predictor of relative dominance rank from childhood through middle adolescence, it is during adolescence that sexual maturation first becomes instrumental in predicting status. Sade (1967) has pointed this out for primate males:

I speculate that at about puberty physiological differences betweeen males become more important in fighting and that the differences that derive from past experiences and continued association with adults of different rank becomes less overriding in determining the winner of fights. (p. 133)

During pubescence sexual dimorphism becomes most pronounced, separating the "men from the women"; during preadolescence both sexes tend to look alike (Freedman, 1979). Counter to Darwin's (1872) belief that secondary sex characteristics evolved as sexual lures, Guthrie (1970) views them as having evolved as social signals, functioning as threat displays to intimidate or antagonize other males after pubescence. For example, the genital area, undergoing radical changes during pubescence, may serve as a social signal. Pubic and auxillary hair function not only as visual displays, but also as olfactory signals of threat. Pubic hair, a darkened scrotum, and enlarged testes and penis are visible signs of a male's approaching maturity, and hence signify to adult males that one is now potentially a sexual and status competitor (Wickler, 1967). In some primate species there is a direct relationship between the progress of pubescent development and the amount of male aggression that one receives (Savin-Williams, in press).

Thus, for primate adolescent males the connection between physical maturation and dominance rank has been theoretically and empirically made. Due to vast deficiencies in studies of primate adolescent females within a group setting, it is not clear what role pubescence has for female adolescent status. Perhaps female secondary sex characters also serve as threat displays among same-sex peers. Or, they may be held in awe or high esteem because of their role as sexual attractants.

Age Trends in Social-Sports Behavior

It was not so much the frequency of social interactions that varied in accordance with the age of the players, but the kind of behavior that was elicited in the two studies of volleyball games. When the participants were early adolescents the frequency of physical contact, teasing, screaming, boasting, and criticism rose precipitously. Enthusiasm for the game through extroverted, perhaps impulsive, behavior was clearly expressed. In their enthusiasm for the game 6th grade girls resembled early adolescent 8th grade boys: The games were emotionally electrifying, frequently chaotic, and certainly noisy. But, after early adolescence the sexes diverged in their approach to volleyball games. Middle adolescent boys became more disciplined, planning strategy, organizing, encouraging fellow teammates, and criticizing each other less frequently. Middle adolescent girls, on the other hand, disassociated themselves from the game, as noted in the increase in distracting activities and the diminished rate of encouraging their peers.

Females

The middle adolescent girls appeared to do everything within their power to deemphasize the game; they engaged in talk about irrelevant events or items, preened themselves (especially concerned about their hair), and avoided the ball if it came toward them.

Originally, I thought the behavioral difference between early and middle adolescent girls would be mirrored in their internalized sex-role orientation. But the degree of masculinity or femininity that a girl expressed on the BSRI did not explain much of these age effects. Uncertain, however, is whether this failure to account for the age difference in social interactions is real or due to problems arising from using the BRSI with this age group. Many of the girls had difficulty understanding several of the adjectives on the BSRI. Thus, it may be that the BSRI is not an appropriate measure to assess degree of masculinity and femininity among early and middle adolescent girls. This issue in self-report research on adolescent populations is frequently ignored, although it may be quite influential. Behavioral research obviously avoids this problem: if the "subject" adequately comprehends the assigned self-report task. This issue will be further explored in Chapter 10.

It is unclear if the age differences noted in this study are developmental differences; to ascertain this one would need a longitudinal research design. Perhaps the age differences are attributable to cohort effects, but I do not think so because it is difficult to imagine that such influences occurred in the two years between the 6th and 8th grade girls and not between the 8th and 10th grade participants. Neither are the differences due to school effects, because the 8th and 10th grade girls were from different schools, and school structures, and yet they were nearly identical in behavioral responses to volleyball games. Rather, I believe the differences are due to influences that affect an early pubescent girl but not a late- or post-pubescent girl.

The introduction to this study of female volleyball games outlines the potentiality of socialization inducers on adolescent girls to behave in a more "lady-like" manner, especially after pubescence. Thus, it is incumbent, it would seem, for the middle adolescent girl to do everything within her power to deemphasize her interest in the masculine pastime of sports, or for that matter, anything she feels is masculine, such as excelling in math and science in high school. The early adolescent girl, on the other hand, may feel less social pressure to deny her involvement and enthusiasm for physical activity. These are, of course, only speculations; uncertain are not only the causal factors (the degree of biological and socialization influences), but also the extent to which the girls' behavior reflects their biological or their socially conditioned state. With the increasing range and flexibility of possible behavioral responses to sports available to adolescent girls today, answers may more likely be forthcoming as to the relative influences of biological and socialization processes on female adolescent behavior.

Males

The findings for males are similar to those on dominance relations in adolescence: Early adolescents were more apt than middle and late adolescents to be physical and overt when dominating camp mates. The subjective impressions of the observers confirmed this basic age difference in the volleyball games. Tenth-grade games appeared more organized, and time-outs were called so strategy could be planned. It was not uncommon to have a "hush" during critical points. This was seldom observed in early adolescent games. When errors were made, early adolescents criticized each other. When plays were good, they congratulated each other physically rather than verbally. Tenth-grade games appeared mentally intense and organized; 8th grade games were emotionally intense and chaotic.

Success situations within the male groups were conducive to positive and harmonious social interactions, on both a verbal and physical level. Failure, however, frequently resulted in either intrateam, not to mention interteam, bickering or a "who-gives-a-damn-its-only-a-game" philosophy. Tied games represented a unique situation, introducing an intense level of competitiveness and an increased frequency of emotional and impulsive social interactions. When an 8th grade score was tied late in a male volleyball game, the observers frequently felt that total anarchy could not be far behind.

Females and Males

Although age remains a significant predictor of social sports behavior among both adolescent males and females, it is not clear what it is about age that is important in influencing social interactions. If it is possible to delineate the causal factors, it may be necessary to explore two components associated with pubescence and adolescence: (1) physiological and biochemical changes that predispose an individual to respond in particular ways to the physical and social environment and (2) socialization processes associated with behaving in socially appropriate or inappropriate ways.

The former is an infrequent concern of developmental psychologists; thus, there is little empirical evidence to suggest possible factors that might be influential. Perhaps there are behavioral consequences of a particular biochemical (male as opposed to female hormonal ratio) or anatomical (strength or size) make-up. Or, the critical consequences of increased advancement in pubescence may revolve around personal and cultural reactions to a changing biology. Looking more like an adult woman may influence the middle adolescent girl to act in a more culturally prescribed feminine fashion.

These studies do not lend assistance to these issues. They do, however, demonstrate age differences in naturally occurring behavior of adolescent girls and boys—an all too rare event in developmental psychology. Because of the exploratory nature of the present investigations and the small sample size, conclusions are necessarily limited. Replication with other populations and during various sports activities are important extensions. This research supplements the infancy of a new science of adolescence psychology that I am advocating because of its documentation of human behavior in real-life settings, and not just where the psychologist finds it convenient to study it.

8
Adolescent Altruism

In addition to competing with each other for status, adolescents also cooperate with each other in altruistic or prosocial behavior. In the two studies described in this chapter, R. Zeldin (RZ) and S. Small (SS) served as observers and co-authors in an investigation of prosocial behavior among adolescent males and females during two summer outcamping trips.

Altruism

In many primate species an individual spends an increasing amount of time with peers as he or she begins pubescence, providing an opportunity to learn a diversified set of roles, skills, and relationships and to develop independence from parents, thus enhancing gene pool dispersion (Hartup, 1983; Savin-Willims, in press; Weisfeld & Berger, 1983). One important dimension of peer group social interactions has been operationalized to encompass a variety of behaviors, such as helping, sharing, rescuing, and comforting, that reflects a concern for others and an adherence to the norm of social responsibility. Social scientists have conducted a number of studies exploring antecedents and correlates of "prosocial" or "altruistic" behavior—but only rarely, however, have they been explored outside of the laboratory.

Several extensive reviews of the prosocial literature have been published that organize the available research into a developmental framework with a focus on the socializing experiences that promote the growth of the altruistic person (Mussen & Eisenberg-Berg, 1977; Radke-Yarrow, Zahn-Waxler, & Chapman, 1983; Rushton, 1980; Staub, 1979). Prosocial behavior is considered to be an essential activity for the effective functioning of social groups, the well-being of society in general (Rushton, 1980), and the survival of the species (Dawkins, 1976; Trivers, 1971). The reviewers note two limitations of this research. First, knowledge of prosocial development is limited to studies of children and adults; most neglect altruism during adolescence, although from a life course perspective experiences occurring after childhood affect patterns of prosocial behavior in adulthood. Second, the reviewers stress a need for research strategies examining altruism in natural settings. Yet, laboratory-based research continues to be the primary means for gathering data among social scientists. The need for empirical research in naturalistic settings is particularly salient in light of Bryan's (1975) suggestion that an individual's altruistic activities may differ depending on whether one is with peers in natural settings or in a laboratory setting with an unfamiliar adult or an anonymous other in need.

Another central issue in the prosocial literature concerns sex differences in helping behavior. Although most studies have not reported consistent patterns of sex differences in altruism (Maccoby & Jacklin, 1974; Radke-Yarrow et al., 1983), generalizations of these preadolescent findings to adolescent populations may be inappropriate due to the significant physical and endocrinological changes of pubescence that alter behavior thresholds and sensitivities (Katchadourian, 1977; Tanner, 1962). Increased societal pressure to behave in a sexually appropriate manner, especially when with peers (Katz, 1979), provides additional impetus for distinctions between the sexes in social behavior. These factors have led Block (1976) to suggest that it is unreasonable to expect sex differences in children's altruism, but studies based on adolescent populations might reveal such differences.

In the present two studies the altruistic activities of adolescent females and males are documented as they occur within the peer group. Extensive observations of spontaneous prosocial behavior were conducted during outcamping trips by RZ and SS, who acted as participant observers. Five questions directed the research:

1. Do members of the peer group perceive individual differences in altruism that are consistent with behavioral differences?
2. How often do adolescents help each other when left to their own resources?
3. What forms of altruism do adolescents initiate?
4. Do the sexes differ in their frequency and form of prosocial behavior?
5. Does the sex of the beneficiary affect the actor's frequency and form of prosocial behavior?

Study One[1]

Setting and Participants

Participants were 12 adolescent males (mean age, 15.5 years, range 14-16 years) attending a five-week wilderness travel program sponsored by

---

[1]This study is based on an article by Zeldin, Savin-Williams, and Small, 1984.

Camp Wancaooah. The boys were from Caucasian, Protestant, two-parent families engaged in professional or managerial occupations. The boys averaged 70 inches in height, 140 pounds in weight, and stage 4 on Tanner's Pubertal Maturational Scale (1962). Prior to camp they were randomly assigned by camp administrators to one of two independent travel groups. Both Group A and Group B consisted of six adolescents each led by a counselor (RZ or SS).

The program consisted of a six-day in-camp training period, a 12-day canoe trip through Ontario, a 12-day bicylce trip through Northern Michigan, and a three-day evaluation period at the base camp. On the first day of camp the boys were asked to participate in a study exploring how groups behave in wilderness settings away from the luxuries of home. All agreed to participate with the assurance of individual feedback and a small financial renumeration.

Measures

Altruism was operationally defined as behavior that met three criteria: (a) the act benefited another individual(s) or group; (b) the actor was not fulfilling any explicitly defined role obligation (e.g., if one's assigned chore on a given day was to make dinner the act was not coded as prosocial, but, if the participant was not assigned this task and he did help, then the act was coded as prosocial); and (c) the behavior of the actor was not solicited by another individual (if an individual was asked to assist another then the act was not coded as prosocial).

After extensive precamp observations of adolescents in various natural settings, five forms of altruism were delineated. Similar to Zahn-Waxler, Radke-Yarrow, and King (1979) and Strayer, Wareing, and Rushton (1979), both verbal and physical forms were included (X denotes the actor):

1. Physical assistance: a nonverbal behavior that provides physical assistance or aid-giving by helping an individual(s) accomplish a definite end. X helps Y set up his tent by hammering the tent stakes.
2. Physical serving: a physical act that benefits another individual(s) and in which the beneficiary(s) does not participate. X fixes the flat tire on Y's bicycle without Y's participation in the task.
3. Sharing: physically giving one's food or possessions to another individual(s). X gives Y an apple.
4. Verbal assistance: a verbal explanation or instruction that assists an indivdual(s) in the performance of a task. X instructs Y how to put up his tent.
5. Verbal support: verbally expressing a concern for reducing the discomfort of a destressed individual(s) in the manner of sympathy, praise, or encouragment. X compliments Y on his cooking ability after others have criticized it.

Because the focus of the study was also to examine the recipients of helping behavior, three "beneficiary" categories were defined:

1. Peer(s): one or two trip members who directly profit from a single act
2. Group: the group as a collective (three or more individuals) who benefit from an act
3. Counselor: the counselor who is helped by a single act.

Observational Method

A time sampling technique was employed in which all occurrences of prosocial behavior were recorded within a limited time span (Wright, 1960). Observations were conducted in three activity settings: group, free time, and individual. Group activities were those in which all participants were in close proximity to one another and engaged in task-oriented activities (e.g., camp set up, meal preparation). Free time involved periods when participants were given a choice in their activities (e.g., discussion, reading). These activity settings were chosen because they were also the counselor's free time; observations could be conducted unhindered by leader responsibilities. Observations averaged a total of .75 hours per day during group activities and .75 hours during free time. If a group member left the observer's view, coding stopped until he returned. Individual activities were those in which the entire group was not present, typically during bicycling, canoeing, hiking, and resting. Each day the counselor chose two individuals, on a rotating basis, to be the focus of observations during individual activities. Over the duration of the trip each camper was observed an average of .40 hours per day during these activities.[2]

When a target behavior was observed, the counselor noted it on a preprinted coding form. Recorded were the date, actor, form of act, beneficiary of act, and the activity in which the act occurred. This direct but unobtrusive method was possible because the youth were aware that the counselor was required by the camp administration to keep a detailed journal of the trip.

Peer Rankings

Four days after the beginning of camp and three day before the end of the camp session, the 12 adolescents completed altruism rankings in

---

[2] Given the nature of the travel programs that involved one group and its counselors being isolated from others, reliability cross-checks were conducted among the three of us at another camp for adolescents that also stressed outdoor activities. During 3.9 hours of observations during canoeing, athletic games, and craft periods, inter-observer agreement averaged .89 (range: .86 to .92). Inter-observer reliabilities for form categories averaged .83 (range: .72 to .94). All reliabilities are based on the percent of agreement of observed episodes.

individual sessions. Each was asked to rank order individuals in his group according to "Who is the most helpful or cooperative in the group?" Composite prosocial hierarchies were derived for each group by averaging the individual orderings. In order to mask the importance of this question, the boys were also asked to rank their peers on the dimensions of self-esteem, dominance, friendship, and camping ability.

Nature of Adolescent Altruism

Table 8.1 presents the distribution of naturally occurring altruism in the two travel groups. The absolute difference in frequency between the groups was not significant[3] and group comparisons across the three dimensions of altruism (form, beneficiary, activity) yielded similar trends. The only noticeable difference was within the form dimension. The boys in Group A initiated verbal assistance more than they did verbal support. The opposite trend was evident in Group B.

Combing the two groups, 377 altruistic acts were observed, an average of 31.4 per participant. Sixty-four percent of the prosocial acts were performed physically, 22% were verbal, and 14% of the acts involved sharing behavior. Altruism was directed about equally to peers, the group, and the counselor and was initiated most frequently in group activities.

In order to provide a summary of the degree of association among the five forms of prosocial behavior, the groups were combined and intercorrelations between individual frequencies of prosocial forms were determined. Of the 10 possible intercorrelations, all were positive and seven were significant. On the basis of overall frequency, participants ranked significantly the same regardless of the form of altruism.[4] Thus, for purposes of this study, the five forms were aggregated into a single measure of altruism.

Individual Consistency in Altruism

To assess the extent that the youth maintained interindividual differences in their frequency of prosocial initiation over time, individual rates were calculated separately for the three phases of the wilderness trip. Correlations between time periods were highly positive, ranging from .84 to .93, all significant to the .005 level. Similarly, high behavioral stability was demonstrated across the three activity settings with a range of correlations between .67 and .96, all significant to the .005 level. Thus, adolescents who were altruistic in one setting and during one time period

---

[3]$t = 1.05$, $df = 10$, ns
[4]$W = .85$, $p < .01$

Table 8.1. Summary of Observed Prosocial Behavior for Two Travel Groups

	Group A (N = 6)		Group B (N = 6)		All Participants (N = 12)	
	Observed frequency	Percent of total behaviors	Observed frequency	Percent of total behaviors	Observed frequency	Percent of total behaviors
I Overall acts	212		165		377	
II Form of altruism						
a) verbal support	13	6%	21	13%	34	9%
b) verbal assistance	35	16%	15	9%	50	13%
c) physical assistance	62	29%	54	33%	116	31%
d) physical serving	73	34%	53	32%	126	33%
e) sharing	31	15%	22	13%	53	14%
III Beneficiary of act						
a) peer	69	33%	60	36%	129	34%
b) group	85	40%	58	35%	143	38%
c) counselor	58	27%	47	29%	105	28%
IV Activity of act						
a) group	99	47%	81	49%	180	48%
b) individual	72	34%	53	32%	125	33%
c) free time	41	19%	31	19%	72	19%

also demonstrated the highest frequency of prosocial behavior in the other two settings and time periods.

Based on the absolute number of acts performed by an individual, a median split was used to separate the high and low helpers. The six individuals who performed the greatest number of prosocial acts (range 31 to 80) were categorized as high helpers (mean, 49.8 acts); the six participants with the lowest rate of helping (range 9 to 16), as low helpers (mean, 13.0 acts). The difference between high and low helpers was significant.[5] Three participants from each travel group were included, via the median split, into both categories of helpers.

Peer Rankings

The group altruism rankings were determined twice, on Day 4 at the end of the training period, and on Day 30 when the participants returned to the base camp. Prosocial hierarchies were derived by averaging the individual rank orderings, including self rankings, of the boys. In both groups, there was a significant intragroup agreement on relative rank at the beginning of the wilderness trip.[6]

Moreover, the basic outline of the peer helping hierarchies remained stable throughout camp. The first and last week helping rank orders were significantly similar in both groups with correlations of .77 and .83. Group helping hierarchies based on the absolute frequency of observed prosocial acts were highly correlated (.92 and .89) with the peer rankings obtained at the end of the trip. Altruistic individuals were clearly recognized by their peers after four days of camp; these perceptions remained consistent over a month; and the peer perceptions agreed with the data obtained from the observational method, demonstrating convergent validity between these two methods.

High and Low Helpers

The absolute and relative frequencies across the three dimensions of prosocial activity for the high and low helpers are presented in Table 8.2. Although the two groups did not differ in the form of altruism initiated, large differences were evident in the beneficiary and activity dimensions. Next, we determined whether the observed frequencies of the beneficiary categories might be expected by chance. The significant result[7] demonstrates that there was an association between the categories of helpers (low, high) and the beneficiaries (group, peer, counselor). When low helpers initiated a prosocial act, it typically benefited the adult counselor

---

[5]$t = 4.66, df = 10, p < .001$
[6]Group A, $W = .50$ and $.59, p < .01$; Group B, $W = .44$ and $.52, p < .05$
[7]$x^2 = 24.29, df = 2, p < .001$

TABLE 8.2. Comparison Between High and Low Helpers

	High helpers (N = 6)		Low helpers (N = 6)	
	Overall frequency	Percent of total behavior	Overall frequency	Percent of total behavior
I Overall acts	299	100%	78	100%
II Form of altruism				
a) verbal support	30	10%	3	4%
b) verbal assistance	40	13%	10	13%
c) physical assistance	89	30%	27	35%
d) physical serving	101	34%	25	31%
e) sharing	39	13%	13	17%
III Beneficiary of act				
a) peer	98	33%	31	39%
b) group	131	44%	12	16%
c) counselor	70	23%	35	45%
IV Activity of act				
a) group	153	51%	27	35%
b) individual	84	28%	41	52%
c) free time	62	21%	10	13%

or a peer. Few of their altruistic acts were directed toward the group. By comparison, the acts of the high helpers benefited the group more frequently than they did peers or the counselor.

We then explored whether high and low helpers differed in the types of activities (group, individual, free time) in which altruistic behavior was performed. The difference was significant,[8] suggesting that prosocial acts occurring during a particular activity differed in the two helper groups. Altruism among low helpers was most frequent during individual activities; high helpers, however, engaged in altruism more during group activities than during individual or free time activities.

Study Two[9]

Setting and Participants

Participants were in one of two groups, on a coed, three-week bicycle trip sponsored by a private youth organization (not Camp Wancaooah). The adolescents, mean age of 15.6 years, were from Caucasian, two-parent

[8] $x^2 = 16.75, df = 2, p < .001$
[9] This study is based on a previously published article (Zeldin, Small, & Savin-Williams, 1982).

families engaged in professional or managerial occupations. Prior to the trip, the youth were randomly assigned by a program adminstrator to one of two travel groups. One group was composed of four females and five males and the other had four females and six males. None of the participants were previously acquainted with other group members. Each group was led by an adult counselor (RZ or SS), and followed identical intineraries through the backroads of northern New England one week apart.

Primary responsibility for the group's functioning was assumed by the adolescents. All group decisions were enacted after consensus was reached among participants; the counselor's principle role was that of a resource person. Each adolescent was informed that the general purpose of the research was to explore how youth interacted in wilderness settings. All chose to participate in the research.

Methods

Altruism was defined, operationalized, and assessed as in Study One. Observations were conducted only when all youth were both visible and audible to the observer (e.g., camp set up and take down, meal preparation, group planning sessions, and free time periods following meals). In addition, observations were conducted during the counselor's free time, periods when campers were aware that they had sole responsibility for the group's functioning. Due to the dual responsibilities of counselor and participant observer, it was decided prior to the trip to limit observations to no more than two hours per day (the two groups averaged 1.37 and 1.70 hours of observation per day).

When a target behavior was observed, the counselor noted it in a journal within 15 minutes of its occurrence. The observer's role as both participant and observer facilitated the ability to observe and collect data on group interactions.

Individual Differences in Altruism

On Day 4 and Day 21 participants ranked members of their travel group from most to least helpful. In both groups there was significant intragroup agreement on relative rank, both at the beginning and at the end of the camping trip.[10] The composite rankings obtained at the beginning of the trip were significantly similar in both groups to those at the end of camp with correlations of .91 and .85. Thus, individual differences in altruism were recognized by peers after only four days of being together, and these perceptions remained stable over a three-week period.

---

[10]$W = .40$ and $.50; p < .05; W = .47$ and $.57; p < .05$

TABLE 8.3. Mean Frequencies of Altruism Across Five Forms of Behavior

	Verbal support	Verbal assistance	Physical serving	Physical assistance	Sharing
Females (N = 8)					
Percent of					
Total Acts	30%	10%	40%	10%	8%
Mean per person	8.62	2.62	10.50	2.75	2.00
Group Mean = 26.49					
Males (N = 11)					
Percent of					
Total Acts	9%	5%	37%	32%	17%
Mean per person	2.36	1.36	10.00	8.36	4.72
Group Mean = 26.80					
All Participants (N = 19)					
Percent of					
Total Acts	20%	7%	38%	22%	13%
Mean per person	5.00	1.89	10.21	6.00	3.58
Group Mean = 26.68					

Behavioral altruism hierarchies were derived at the trip's completion by summing the number of acts observed for each adolescent and ordering individuals according to their frequency of prosocial behavior. The frequency range in Group A was 9 to 46 prosocial acts and in Group B the range was 12 to 63 acts. Behavioral hierarchies correlated (.79 and .94) highly with the last week composite altruism peer rankings, demonstrating convergent validity between the two methods.

Comparison by Sex Across Prosocial Activity

In Group A, 211 total acts were observed over 28.75 hours and in Group B, 296 acts were recorded during 35.65 hours. Individuals averaged .76 prosocial acts per hour in the former group and .92 in the latter. Table 8.3 presents summary data for the five forms of altruism separate by sex.

Patterns of altruism were examined by computing the total number of behaviors observed for each of the 19 participants across the five prosocial form categories. There were no main effects for group or sex, demonstrating no difference in the frequency of altruism between the two groups or between boys and girls, but the main effect for prosocial form was significant.[11] Post-hoc paired comparisons indicated significant differences betweeen physical serving and the other form categories and

---

[11]$F(4, 94) = 8.44$; $p < .001$. Because Group B was observed slightly more than Group A, the groups were weighted by mulitplying the behavioral observations in Group B by the value .86 (total observation time in Group A divided by the total observation time in Group B).

TABLE 8.4. Mean Frequencies of Altruism Across Three Categories of Beneficiary

	Peers	Group	Counselors
Females (N = 8)			
Percent of total acts	48%	39%	13%
Mean per person	13.50	10.75	3.50
Group Mean = 27.75			
Males (N = 11)			
Percent of total acts	45%	37%	18%
Mean per person	12.45	10.45	5.00
Group Mean = 27.90			
All participants (N = 19)			
Percent of total acts	46%	38%	16%
Mean per person	12.89	10.58	4.36
Group Mean = 27.83[a]			

[a]Means are greater than in Table 8.3 because a small number of single prosocial acts (N = 22) benefited both a peer and counselor.

between physical serving, physical assistance, and verbal support and the categories of sharing and verbal assistance.

The group x sex interaction was also significant.[12] In Group A, females averaged 1.04 altruistic acts per hour and males averaged .53. In Group B, the males averaged 1.14 acts per hour compared to the females' mean of .64. The group x form interaction was not significant.

Of special interest was the significant interaction between sex and prosocial form.[13] Hierarchical regression runs, with prosocial form as the dependent variable, were conducted to further delineate these effects. Of the five interactions between sex and prosocial form, two were significant: verbal support and physical assistance.[14] In the category of verbal support, females averaged 8.62 acts and males averaged 2.36. By comparison, males averaged 8.36 physical assistance acts compared to the mean of 2.75 for females.

Comparisons by Sex Across Beneficiary Categories

Table 8.4 presents the means for the three beneficiary categories; a main effect for beneficiary was significant.[15] Both sexes had similar patterns in whom they chose to help; males and females were more altruistic toward peers and the group than to the counselor.

To explore same- and mixed-sex altruistic interactions, an analysis was performed on those prosocial acts that benefited either a female or a male

[12] $F(1, 94) = 11.36; p < .001$
[13] $F(4, 94) = 4.26; p < .004$
[14] $F(4, 79) = 5.35; p < .001; F(4, 79) = 9.17, p < .001$
[15] $F(2, 56) = 6.55, p < .003$

TABLE 8.5. Mean Number of Altruistic Acts: Actor × Beneficiary × Form

Actor	Beneficiary	Verbal help[a]	Physical help[b]	Sharing	Total acts
Male	Male	.91	2.64	.45	4.00
	Female	1.72	4.36	1.27	7.35
Female	Male	3.38	1.38	.50	5.26
	Female	4.50	1.38	.38	6.26

[a] verbal assistance and support
[b] physical serve and assistance

peer (Table 8.5). To increase the number of acts per cell, categories were combined: verbal support and verbal assistance ("verbal helping"), physical serving and physical assistance ("physical helping"), and "sharing."

The main effect for sex of beneficiary and all interactions were non-significant. Thus, the sex of the beneficiary did not have an effect on whether different patterns of altruism were initiated by boys or girls.

Comparisons by Sex on Peer Measures

Analysis of peer rankings, collected on Day 21, revealed that in both groups neither sex was portrayed as being the more dominant or the more popular nor as having the higher self-esteem. Boys tended to be perceived as the "most competent" camper.[16] Consistent with behavioral observations of prosocial frequency, there was a trend in Group A for females to be ranked as more "helpful" than their male counterparts; in Group B, males were perceived as being more helpful.[17]

Implications

The adolescent participants initiated a variety of altruistic acts that ranged from comforting a distressed peer to patching another's flat tire; the majority were physical serving and physical assistance. The youth varied in their frequency of prosocial behavior; simply, some initiated many acts while others rarely helped. Within days of group formation individual differences were clearly recognized by group members as demonstrated by the strong intragroup agreements in prosocial rank orderings, and the convergence between peer rankings and behaviorally

[16] $t(8) = 1.77$ and $t(7) = 1.90$; p's $< .10$
[17] $t(8) = 2.09$, $p < .06$; $t(7) = 2.25$; $p < .05$

based altruistic measures. The consistency of participants' initiation of prosocial acts during the three or five weeks of camp and across activity settings, along with the significantly high intercorrelations among the five forms of behavior, support the argument that by adolescence some individuals have established a higher level of altruistic behavior than have others.

The smaller number of verbal than physical helping behaviors among the youth was unexpected given the broad definition of the two verbal categories. Moreover, because the youth were exposed to many unique tasks (e.g., orienting with map and compass), there were numerous situations when a verbal act would have been beneficial.

The data indicate that characteristics of the beneficiaries did not differentially affect the decisions of boys and girls to help. Both sexes performed a high percentage of acts that benefited the group. These acts were usually necessary for maintaining the group's day-to-day functioning (e.g., preparing meals, cleaning the campsite), but were rarely assigned by the counselor because the campers volunteered to perform them. The sexes demonstrated equal concern for the group as a collective. Similar findings are evident in the analysis of peer-directed altruistic behavior. Given the heightened importance of sexual relations during adolescence, it was surprising that the sex of the beneficiary was not related to the frequency or form of altruistic behavior. The relatively high number of acts that benefited the single adult counselor was also unexpected. Often, when the counselor was sitting apart from the group enjoying his free time, participants went out of their way to assist or to share food. This suggests that the age or status of the beneficiary may have a powerful impact on the frequency of adolescent altruistic behavior.

The decision to act in an altruistic manner is not independent of the immediate social and physical contexts. Both high and low helpers in Study One demonstrated a degree of specificity in whom they helped. The low helpers directed 45% of their total prosocial acts toward the single adult counselor, but only 8% toward the group. This difference becomes more pronounced when one considers that there were many more opportunities to help the group (e.g., prepare dinner, clean campsite) than to help the counselor. By comparison, the high helper was most likely to respond to group needs and less frequently directed altruistic behavior toward the counselor. Thus, situations necessitating group-oriented action appeared to inhibit the low helpers' performance of altruism while the same situations promoted helping behaviors by those in the high helper group.

Response specificity by the low helpers was also apparent in the activities in which they chose to help. Even though observations were twice as frequent during group activites, over one-half of the low helpers' altruistic acts were initiated during individual activities. High helpers were more consistent with probability expectations, performing most of their prosocial acts during group activities. Perhaps low helpers, when in a situation where the entire group was present, felt little obligation to assist because others were present who could provide the necessary help. This interpretation is consistent with the findings of Latane and Darley (1970) who reported that the number of persons present in a situation strongly affects the likelihood that an individual will choose to help. Specifically, individuals are less likely to help as the number of potential helpers increases. Little is known, however, about the characteristics of those who do help. It is conceivable that high helpers in the present study were those who would help regardless of how many others were present. Similarly, because others were present, the low helpers might have been those who perceived the situation as one not needing their participation, and, subsequently, decided to ignore the individual in need of assistance.

The findings on altruism parallel the results on dominance behavior. Similar to past research with children, individual variation in altruism was not systematically related to sex, thus substantiating Maccoby and Jacklin's (1974) conclusion that neither sex should be considered more altruistic. The sexes did vary, however, on mode of altruism.

Although the two independent bicycle groups displayed divergent rates between males and females in helping peers, the sex differences in forms of prosocial expression remained the same in both groups. When a potential beneficiary was in need of comforting, females were more likely to offer help than were males. In comparison, males were more responsive when the situation offered the opportunity for physical assistance. Although it was the observers' impression that males and females did not differ in their camping abilities, trends consistent with sex-role stereotypes were found in the bicycle groups for the males to be perceived as the more competent campers. In tasks requiring physical assistance, perhaps males took the initiative, or the females deferred because of this shared perception of competance. An entry from the observer's journal illustrates these differences:

Kelly was adjusting the brakes on her bicycle. A taut cable broke and struck her in the face. Kelly fell back, apparently in pain. Without hesitation, Joan ran over and comforted her. A couple of minutes later, Jane walked over, put her arm around Kelly and asked if she was feeling better. The boys in the group continued to work as if nothing had happened. Ten minutes later Kelly returned to work on her bicycle. Edgar, noticing that she was having difficulty, walked over and assisted her in replacing the cable.

These sex differences are contrary to findings with young children (Eisenberg-Berg & Lennon, 1980; Hartup & Keller, 1960; Whiting & Edwards, 1973; Yarrow, Waxler, and associates, 1976), but they are consistent with sex differences in dominance behavior.

To the popular mind altruism and dominance are frequently thought to be inversely related. Altruism is cooperative; dominance is competitive. The former is a hallmark of socialism while the latter is central to capitalism. The prosocial person is a friend to all, kind, considerate, and, perhaps, feminine. The dominant individual, on the other hand, is a leader, powerful, influential, and, perhaps, masculine. On the other hand, Esser (1973) projects altruistic behavior as an alternative mental schemata to accomplish social order.

Results from Study One and Two, summarized in Table 9.5, contradict the popular mind. Correlations in all four groups between altruism and dominance, regardless of the method of assessment, were low and positive—and not significant in a negative direction—averaging .29 and .20 for observations and peer rankings, respectively, Thus, altruism and dominance share some amount of variance. The manner in which the two were defined in the present series of studies, however, accounts for this. For example, a prosocial act such as praising another is also a behavior recognizing the dominance status of the other; the altruistic act of giving unsolicited advice or suggestions is also an act of dominance.

The present studies, describing patterns of adolescent altruistic behavior, demonstrate that both characteristics of the individual and of the social context contribute to the expression of prosocial behavior. There is evidence for an altruistic trait and for the position that situations influence the expression of altruism. It is important that future research examine both sides of the person-situation interaction. These will be discussed further in Chapter 9.

9
Dominance and Altruism as Traits

Introduction

One issue in psychology that persists despite frequent, incontrovertible research studies that purport to close the final curtain, is whether, and to what degree, various personality attributes are traits or states. If trait, then individuals will differ from one another on certain behavioral dimensions and these differences will be relatively stable over time and across settings; if state, then individuals will vary differentially in their behavioral response depending on any number of variables, such as physical setting, social context, and who else is present. The controversy arose in response to the lack of empirical evidence demonstrating the cross-situational consistency of observed behavior. This failure led some personality researchers to question the theoretical utility of the trait concept (Mischel, 1968), or to suggest a reformulation of the traditional conceptualization of "personality trait" (Alker, 1972; Bowers, 1973). One recent resolution to this dilemma has been to propose a person-situation, interactional psychology of personality (Endler, 1975; Endler & Magnusson, 1976). But there are still strong arguments for a trait approach (Buss & Craik, 1980; Buss & Plomin, 1984; Epstein, 1979 & 1980).

These issues are of far more concern to developmental psychologists than to human ethologists; it would be a rare ethologist who would deny the existence of relatively stable individual attributes that are manifested in social interactions. The objection raised by Bernstein (1981) in his summary paper, however, is just this issue. He maintained that dominance is frequently used as a characteristic of an individual when, in reality, it connotes a relationship state, not a trait. Several commentators disagreed; these views are discussed more fully in Chapter 2.

Given the history of the *psychology* of adolescence, the focus has traditionally been on the state of adolescence and seldom on the behavioral traits[1] that precede and succeed adolescence.

---

[1]Here I disagree with the assessments made by reviewers of the research agendas for adolescence cited in Chapter 1 (Berzonsky, 1983; Blyth, 1983; Hill, 1983).

In sum, a strong case for adolescence must deal squarely with the two-sided contention that adolescence makes no specific or lasting contribution to personality, because, first, it is weak against the much larger thrust of behavioral stabilities over the early life span; second, the sound and fury that distinguish it also extinguish it, leaving little of conceptual importance. (Livson & Peskin, 1980; p. 70)

Livson and Peskin (1980) suggest that what may appear to be phenotypically dissimilar traits over time may actually be one genotypically continuous characteristic; thus, it may be more profitable to pursue underlying patterns of behavior that assume different forms over the life course rather than to search for stability in a particular feature. For example, the early maturing male may appear "healthy" in adolescence, but his conformity to social convention may manifest itself in adulthood as poor psychological health because the underlying characteristic of social conformity that appears to others to be healthy during adolescence ("He's so mature!") does not during adulthood ("He's so inflexible!").

Both competitiveness and cooperativeness have received support from the trait and state schools. These issues are briefly discussed before research is described that directly assesses the degree to which dominance and altruism are states, dependent on the social context, or traits, stable characteristics of the individual.

Altruism

Reviewers of the prosocial literature who have theorized the existence of an altruistic trait (Mussen & Eisenberg-Berg, 1977; Rushton, 1980; Staub, 1978 & 1979) have noted the lack of evidence that bears on the issue. Mussen and Eisenberg-Berg (1977) summarize this position:

... a number of other investigations have demonstrated the generality of prosocial behavior, discovering predominantly positive and significant, although not always high, correlations among prosocial measures. This is especially true when these measures are based on natural observations or situations, and global indices (indices composed of several measures). Assessments derived from confined, artificial situations such as highly limited situational tests are less frequently found to correlate with other indices. (p. 19)

Those who have failed to find evidence for a prosocial trait tend to correlate single behavioral measures (e.g., Hartshorne, May, & Maller, 1929)—an insufficient sample size of behavior required by the trait concept. By contrast, those who have reported evidence for the generality of altruism (i.e., traits) employ global or aggregated measures of repeated observations (e.g., Burton's, 1963, reanalysis of Hartshorne et. al., 1929; Friedrich & Stein, 1973) or measures based on peer or teacher ratings (e.g., Dlugokinski & Firestone, 1973).

Dominance

Vaughn and Waters (1980) suggest that within a group, dominance relations form and remain relatively stable because they are the result of unique, genetic characteristics of group members emerging in interpersonal interactions. Chase (1981) proposes that the primary physiological mechanism underlying dominance is arousal level. Thus, one would expect a high degree of stability in the expression of competitive behavior within a group.

Weisfeld, Omark, and Cronin (1980) reported that Omark and Edelman's (1976) first and third grade children maintained their relative dominance positions years later as high school freshman and at high school graduation (Weisfeld, Muczenski, Weisfeld, & Omark, in preparation). With peer ratings Olweus (1977) found a high degree of individual stability among 13 year old boys over one and three year intervals in "aggression"—a term defined similarly to several of the Camp Wancaooah indices of dominance: starts fights with peers, other boys at school tease him, and when a teacher criticizes him he tends to answer back and protest.

Observing Dominance and Altruism

The general issue of whether evidence for personality traits can be found when ethological methods are employed and the more specific issue of whether there is evidence for an altruistic and a dominance trait—that is, are some youth more altruistic or dominant than others and are these differences stable over time and across situations—are pursued here.[2] Naturalistic methodologies that employ extensive observations and multidimensional behavioral definitions provide a research strategy most capable of addressing the trait controversy. To assess the trait properties of altruism and dominance and the effectiveness of the methodologies employed, a multitrait-multimethod framework (Campbell & Fiske, 1959) is modeled. To assess convergent validity two methods of measurement are included: naturalistic observation and peer ratings; to establish divergent validity both dominance and altruism are included as behavioral categories.

Methods

Four groups were observed as they interacted in naturalistic settings. Groups 1 and 2 are Study One participants reported in Chapter 8. In

---

[2] The research is reported more completely in Small, Savin-Williams, & Zeldin, 1983.

addition to the observations and peer rankings of altruism described in Chapter 8, dominance interactions were assessed. Congruent with the earlier Camp Wancaooah studies, the same eight indices of behavior were used as measures of dominance. I observed dominance interactions in each group during the nine in-camp days and RZ or SS, the group camp counselors, observed the same during the 24 out-of-camp days. Prior to camp RZ and SS were familiarized with the eight types of dominance behaviors and the recording procedures. Their dual role as group counselor and research observer enabled the direct but unob-trusive recording of behavior *in situ.* For example, when the boys were planning their next trip, the counselor noted group interactions in-dicative of dominance. When recording data was not immediately feasible (while bicycling or canoeing), interactions were dictated at the next possible moment, usually within 15 minutes. I was able to record data unobtrusively during the in-camp days because of my role at Camp Wancaooah. As program director, my presence and clipboard were not construed by campers as being unusual or obtrusive.

For an average of 1.5 hours per day during the nine in-camp days and during 22 of the 24 out-of-camp days (omitting the first hectic days of the bicycle and canoe trips), RZ and SS recorded all episodes of dominance behavior that occurred in dyadic interactions between members of the travel group (total hours observed, 93 hours). Observations were made during mealtimes (30 minutes, usually at dinner), group discussions (30 minutes, usually after dinner when talking about the day's activities or after breakfast when planning the day's schedule), and individual activities or free time (30 minutes, during bicycling, canoeing, or repairing bicycles). The 1.5-hour observation time per day was construed by the three of us as being a sufficient compromise between the research need to record normative, natural behavior and the need to be a counselor.

The adolescents in Groups 3 and 4 were the same youth described in Study Two (Chapter 8). In addition to altruism, SS and RZ also recorded instances of the eight indices of dominance for an average of .5 hours per day (during times when altruistic behavior was not being recorded).[3]

In all groups, four days after the beginning of the travel camp session

---

[3]Given the nature of the travel camp programs, which involved the isolation of one group from the other, reliability cross-checks for prosocial and dominance behavior were conducted at another camp setting for adolescents. During eight hours of observations during which observers assumed participant-observer roles, recording all instances of prosocial or dominance behavior, inter-observer agreement among the three authors averaged .83 (range: .81 to .84) for dominance behavior and .89 (range: .86 to .92) for prosocial behavior. Inter-observer reliabilities for form categories averaged .78 (range: .68 to .88) for dominance behavior and .83 (range: .72 to .94) for altruism. All reliability values are based on the percent of agreement in observed episodes.

TABLE 9.1. Concordance Coefficients for Dominance and
Altruism

	Dominance	Altruism
Group 1 (n = 6)	.77**	.85**
Group 2 (n = 6)	.85**	.63**
Group 3 (n = 9)	.58**	.42*
Group 4 (n = 10)	.59**	.69**

*$p < .05$
**$p < .01$

and again three days before the end of the trip, all participants were
interviewed individually. Each youth was asked to rank order others in
his or her group according to "Who is the most helpful or cooperative in
the group?" and "Who displays the most dominance in the group?"
Composite altruism and dominance hierarchies were derived for each
group by averaging individual rank orders. To mask the importance of
these questions, participants were also asked to rank their peers on self-
esteem, popularity, and camping ability.[4]

Examined are those properties commonly proposed as indices of traits:
cross-form stability, temporal stability, and cross-situational stability. To
assess the discriminant and convergent validity of the measures, the data
were also examined within a multitrait-multimethod framework. Most
interpretations of the personality trait concept agree with Alston's (1975)
definition of the frequency concept of dispositions: When a particular
trait is attributed to an individual, then given a representative set of
situations, an individual will display a greater number of responses
relative to the norm for that trait. The frequency concept also implies the
existence of a "category of acts" that are topographically dissimilar, but
are nonetheless considered to be manifestations of a common trait (Buss
& Craik, 1980).

Cross-Form Stability

Congruent with a frequency interpretation of personality traits, in each
group the youths ranked significantly the same on the eight forms of
dominance behavior and the five forms of prosocial behavior (Table 9.1).
That is, those who ranked high on one form of dominance or altruism
also tended to rank high on the other forms of that behavior.

---

[4]Reliability values for peer rankings were determined by comparing rankings
among individuals in each group. Time 1 peer rankings for both dominance and
altruism were significantly similar in seven of eight possible cases, with
correlations ranging from .35 to .73. Similarly, agreements among peers for Time
2 rankings were significant in all eight possible cases (correlations between .49
and .85).

TABLE 9.2. Pearson Correlations for Dominance and Altruism across Three Time Periods

	Dominance			Altruism		
	time 1 × time 2	time 2 × time 3	time 1 × time 3	time 1 × time 2	time 2 × time 3	time 1 × time 3
1 (n = 6)	.94**	.82*	.96**	.89**	.89**	.97**
2 (n = 6)	.95**	.33	.49	.93**	.94**	.93**
3 (n = 9)	.80**	.74**	.77**	.57*	.83**	.83**
4 (n = 10)	.62	.87**	.54*	.90**	.43	.64*

*p < .05
**p < .01

Temporal Stability: Observational Measures

Temporal stability refers to the degree that the youths maintained the same rank order (individual differences) over the course of the trip for a particular target behavior. Stability coefficients were obtained in each group by dividing the camp period into three equal time segments and comparing the behavior for each third. Totals for each third were then correlated with the behavior occurring during the other two time periods. As noted in Table 9.2, temporal stability of dominance and altruism tended to be extremely high across the three time periods in each group. That is, individuals who displayed a high frequency of altruism or dominance relative to other group members at Time One continued to maintain these individual differences over the other two time periods.

Temporal Stability: Peer Rankings

Temporal stability coefficients were also computed for peer rankings. First, composite scores for peer ratings of dominance and altruism were calculated by totaling individual rank orders for the two peer assessment

TABLE 9.3. Pearson Correlations for Peer Rankings of Dominance and Altruism

	Dominance Day 4 × Final Day	Altruism Day 4 × Final Day
Group 1 (n = 6)	.82*	.77*
Group 2 (n = 6)	.98**	.83*
Group 3 (n = 9)	.88**	.85**
Group 4 (n = 10)	.83**	.87**

*p < .05
**p < .01

TABLE 9.4. Pearson Correlations for Observed Behaviors in Three Settings

Settings	Group 1 (n = 6)		Group 2 (n = 6)		Group 3 (n = 9)		Group 4 (n = 10)	
	Pro-social	Domi-nance	Pro-social	Domi-nance	Pro-social	Domi-nance	Pro-social	Domi nance
S1–S2	.99**	.93**	.91**	.95**	.48	.63*	.79**	.89**
S2–S3	.73*	.72*	.85*	.33	.60*	.87**	.92**	.70**
S1–S3	.78*	.76*	.85*	.49	.80**	.79**	.72**	.72**

Note-Setting types: S1 = camping; S2 = meals; S3 = free time
*$p < .05$
**$p < .01$

sessions. These composite scores were then correlated with one another and are presented in Table 9.3. For all groups, peer ratings obtained on Day 4 for both dominance and altruism were significantly similar to the peer perceptions obtained at the end of the trip. In other words, individual differences in altruism and dominance were clearly recognized by peers after only four days and these perceptions remained stable over the course of the trips.

Cross-Situational Stability

To assess the degree of cross-situational stability of prosocial and dominance behavior in each group, observational data for both behaviors were summed separately for each of the three activity settings. Correlation coefficients among these three activity settings for all groups are displayed in Table 9.4. The results demonstrate a high degree of cross-situational stability for both altruism and dominance. Thus, regardless of the situation the youth maintained their rank order relative to other group members on the two behavioral dimensions.

Multitrait-Multimethod Analysis

Campbell and Fiske's (1959) multitrait-multimethod framework is a validation procedure using a matrix of intercorrelations among tests representing at least two traits, each measured by at least two methods. This matrix may be analyzed to evaluate the convergent and discriminant validity of the measures. Convergent validity is demonstrated by the degree to which assessments of the same trait, measured by independent methods, intercorrelate. The extent to which measures of different traits are indexing different dimensions—do not intercorrelate highly—provides the basis for discriminant validity. Based on these criteria, the present data provide evidence consistent with convergent and discriminant validity (Table 9.5).

TABLE 9.5. Multitrait-Multimethod Matrix Summary Table

Group	Monotrait-hetero-method		Heterotrait-mono-method		Heterotrait-hetero-method	
	A1–A2	D1–D2	A1–D1	A2–D2	A1–D2	D1–A2
1 (n = 6)	.62	.77*	.27	.07	.46	.34
2 (n = 6)	.73*	.86*	.42	.15	.25	.16
3 (n = 9)	.76**	.88**	.38	.25	.02	.06
4 (n = 10)	.82**	.88**	.09	.31	.21	.05
average	.73	.85	.29	.20	.24	.15

Note– A1 = altruistic behavior observations; A2 = altruism peer perceptions; D1 = dominance behavior observations; D2 = dominance peer perceptions.
* $p < .05$.
** $p < .01$.

The monotrait-heteromethod Pearson correlations for both dominance and altruism (columns 1 and 2 in Table 9.5) provide clear evidence for convergent validity of the two methods. For seven of the eight correlations, peer perceptions of dominance and altruism were highly and significantly correlated with the independent behavioral observation data. Thus, assessments of the behaviors under study were not biased by a particular method of measurement.

Evidence for the discriminant validity of dominance and altruism is indicated by the low and non-significant heterotrait-monomethod correlations (columns 3 and 4 in Table 9.5). It should also be noted that for dominance and altruism the convergent validity correlations (columns 1 and 2) were clearly higher than corresponding heterotrait-monomethod correlations (columns 3 and 4) in all groups. That is, the same trait assessed by two different methods, correlated much higher than did different behaviors measured by the same method. Finally, the heterotrait-heteromethod correlations (columns 5 and 6) tended on the average to be lower than corresponding heterotrait-monomethod correlations (columns 3 and 4). This is as expected, because different traits measured by the same method should share some common method variance while different traits as assessed by different methods should have little or no method variance in common, consequently lowering heterotrait correlations. Thus, the results of the present study provide evidence consistent with trait conceptions of dominance and altruism.

Dominance and Altruism as Traits

The adoption of a frequency interpretation of traits and the subsequent use of a broad category of acts as indicators of each trait provide a more comprehensive description of behavioral regularities than do measures that are defined by single acts. As Jaccard (1974), Buss and Craik (1980), and Gifford (1982) have argued, the multiple act criteria constitutes the appropriate criteria from a frequency interpretation of personality. The present data support this view: For both dominance and altruism topographically dissimilar but conceptually related forms of each behavior were related.

Traits are useful constructs for describing individual differences when behavior is examined over a number of situations. Thus, if a trait measure is based on behavior averaged over situations, differences between individuals can be accurately predicted in the future when the criteria is an average over a similar behavioral sample. It is important to note that because the present research follows an individual differences paradigm, the data tell us little about the instability or stability of behavior within any one given individual (Lamiell, 1981). What the data do tell us is that within *groups* of adolescents, individuals differ from one another on the dimensions of altruism and dominance and these differences are stable across situations and over time.

Although most personality inventories implicitly adhere to the frequency concept, few observational studies of personality employ methods that measure a range of behaviors on more than one occasion. Yet, extensive behavioral observations are necessary when traits are viewed as actuarial or summary terms that are valid over situations in the aggregate (Cronbach, 1975). This problem becomes salient in light of Epstein's (1979, 1980) argument that a large sample of behavior must be obtained to demonstrate the stability of individual differences and to provide evidence for personality traits. He points out that most behavioral studies of personality are conducted in the laboratory and involve single items of behavior on one occasion. A single sample of behavior, similar to items on a paper and pencil test, has too high a component of error to predict behavioral stability. In order to provide evidence for traits, measurement error must be reduced. Epstein and others suggest that reliability can be enhanced by averaging or aggregating measures of the behavior in question over a large number of occasions. For example, Rushton (Rushton, Brainerd, & Pressley, 1983; Rushton, Chrisjohn, & Fekken, 1981) argues against single, behavioral items and for aggregates, the sum of a set of multiple measurements, that average out errors, thus giving a more accurate picture of a variable in a population. Using such procedures Rushton, Fulker, Neale, Blizard and Eysenck (1984) found sufficient evidence to support the notion of a broad base trait of altruism with a genetic underpinning. From a sample of adult twins, both MZ and DZ pairs, they demonstrated that 50% of the variance on several altruism scales was associated with genetic effects. The remaining 50% could be attributed to each twin's specific environment and to measurement error, but not to the twins' common environment.

   The results of the present study provide evidence consistent with trait conceptions of dominance and altruism. This conclusion is supported by multiple criteria, replicated in four groups that converge in demonstrating validity. First, frequency counts of behavior by trained observers indicated that stable individual differences existed regardless of the situation in which they were observed. Second, there was high agreement among peers in attributing dominance and altruism to individuals with whom they interacted. Third, and perhaps most important, there were substantial positive correlations between observed behavior and peer perceptions. Although these two methods are somewhat similar in that they are both based on the observation of naturally occurring behavior, they are distinct in several ways. The former employed trained observers while the latter did not, and the trained observers limited their observation to brief time periods in specific situations, whereas peer perceptions were derived from more global observations of ongoing interactions. Consequently, the high correspondence between these two methods provides strong evidence for the existence of stable individual differences because these differences were evident not only to the trained observers in the sample of situations in which they observed, but also to the untrained participants in the day-to-day activities in which they interacted. Finally, additional support for the present conclusions are provided by the high temporal stability coefficients. Regardless of the method employed, stable individual differences in altruism and dominance behavior over time were clearly evident.

   If composite scores of helping behavior observed in natural settings are good indices of altruistic dispositions, as suggested by Mussen and Eisenberg-Berg (1977) and Staub (1979), then, by adolescence, stable individual differences in altruism are observed. The same appears true for dominance behavior because of the strong equivalence among the eight forms of dominance behavior, substantiating Buss and Craik's (1980) and Candland and Hoer's (1981) contention that dominance is best measured through constructing mega-categories of related acts.

Dominance

A diversity of behaviors were used by the adolescents in the research reported in this book to assert or recognize relative differences among themselves in status. The eight indices of dominance and submission are not all inclusive of the many ways in which individuals express their power, and neither are they equivalent in content or form but in effect: one individual dominating another. In content, many of the behaviors are also indicative of other constructs. For example, giving advice to another may be an act of friendship as well as an act of dominance.

Hitting a cabinmate may be an act of wild rage or aggression as well as an act connoting relative dominance status.

In form, dominance ranged from overt to subtle, from the hardly detectable to the outrageous, and from vocalizations to physical acts. Individual adolescents varied considerably in their style of expressing status. For example, some adolescents appear to be bullies, physically asserting themselves in a rather overt and aggressive manner. Others display more finesse, using subtle, nonthreatening behaviors such as shunning or ignoring to promote their status. Although the former seems to be the lay person's understanding of dominance, the latter behaviors were usually far more successful strategies in asserting dominance among peers. The power of suggestion may be far more effective than physical aggression in maintaining one's position, even among the savages known as adolescents.

There is nothing contradictory in this diversity, nor should it be surprising. Body parts, and their behaviors, have many functions; for example, the penis serves elimination, reproduction, and status functions. The latter is evident in some forms of early Greek art and among nonhuman primates. Loizos (1969) distinguished play from dominance behavior in chimpanzees by noting that the same motor patterns may have different signal patterns that lead to dispersal (dominance), imitation (play), or a new set of behaviors (either). Given a different context and a slightly different meaning, Weisfeld and Weisfeld (1984) found that praise could be used to assert dominance rather than to serve as an act of submission. Thus, the consequences of behavior are crucial in the labeling process.

Although these behaviors reflect a dominance personality trait, it is also true that different situations elicited different response styles. For example, during athletic games and "rest hour" rough-and-tumble play activities and physical threats were frequent means of expressing dominance; verbal arguments and interruptions were common behaviors during group discussions. An effective alpha knows when and how to express his or her status; behavior adaptation is a mark of power and influence that stabilizes and maintains an adolescent's position at the top. Without it, it is doubtful that he or she would remain most dominant.

Thus, the specific behaviors used to express dominance status may vary by an individual's personality style, the situation in which the act occurs, and one's age or sex (discussed previously). These variations should not, however, disguise the fact that a conceptualization of dominance as a higher order phenomenon than specific behaviors is warranted. In all groups studied, the specific indices of dominance were significantly intercorrelated. That is, although adolescents behaved differently within a group and in various contexts, they maintained the same relative rank regardless of the activity.

Athletic Ability and Dominance

Athletic ability was a consistent predictor of dominance status among the eight groups of early adolescents and the 52 groups of early to middle adolescents in the all-camp study. It is also predictive of relative status at other points in the life course from childhood through adulthood and among youth in other cultures. For example, Zarit (1970) concluded that a dominance hierarchy is based on relative ability in playing games and in fighting among first graders; both rely on somewhat the same traits: strength, speed, coordination, aggressiveness, and self-assurance. This relationship was also confirmed among Hopi and Afro-American grade school children (Weisfeld, Weisfeld, & Callaghan, 1982). Sherif and Sherif (1964) noted in their groups of adolescent boys that the most athletic individuals were also the ones with the most social power. Among West Point male cadets participation in sports correlated with military rank during the college years and at the end of the military career. That is, those who lettered at West Point were "twice as likely as those never on a collegiate team to attain the highest ranks." (Mazur, Mazur, & Keating, 1984; p. 140)

Uncertain, however, is whether the relationship between athletic ability and dominance is due to biological features (physique, strength, coordination, neurological factors) of the athlete, to personal characteristics such as courage or leadership, to the symbolic value of athletic participation, or to all three (Mazur et al., 1984). Weisfeld et al. (in preparation) argue rather convincingly for a genetic explanation. Although enhanced by practice and experience, athletic ability is largely dependent on heritable characteristics such as muscular development, body shape, and aerobic power (Klissouras, 1984). For Weisfeld et al. (in preparation) the constellation of physical traits that are determinants of dominance status also includes physical attractiveness, strength, and early maturity—all of which emerge long before puberty, perhaps with a sensitive period around six years of age. These facts would account for the relative stability of dominance status over the life course. Similarly, pubertal development correlates highly with dominance status not so much because of its social value, as concluded by social learning theorists (Mussen & Jones, 1957), but because of its relation to other physical traits shared with athletic ability and dominance and its signal of reproductive maturity (Weisfeld et al., in preparation).

Athletic ability significantly predicted dominance status in female as well as male adolescent groups; thus, the above male-oriented assertions may also be true for females. This is counter to the speculation of Weisfeld et al. (in preparation) who report that physical traits such as strength, muscularity, and athletic ability do not lead to social success or high status among girls. But, with the increasing participation and visibility of female athletes in tennis, basketball, golf, and track, perhaps adolescent females also accede to those who possess natural coordination that combines physical abilities, strength, assertiveness, and self-assurance. The sparse literature on female adolescent groups and our blindness to the existence of female assertiveness negate the possibility of finding a correspondence between physical prowess and dominance states. These are exactly the points made by the collected work on nonhuman primate female research reported in Small (1984): Most primatological research centers on male dominance and little is understood regarding the nature or correlates of female dominance. Lancaster (1984) reports that female primates have also evolved to be fierce competitors with a concern for status and an ability to be aggressive in achieving it.

Conclusion

Aside from major disruptions, relative dominance status remained stable over time and settings, increasing in stability as group members more clearly distinguished relative status. Challenges became more selective, respecting clearly established dyadic relationships while challenging the flexible ones. This plasticity was prevalent to varying degrees in the adolescent groups, perhaps more so in female groups.

The dominance structure was constant not only temporally, but also situationally. Counter to conventional wisdom that different settings elicit a particular kind of leader, thus implying that dominance status should vary by behavior setting, group members ranked significantly the same regardless of the setting in which they were observed. It might be argued that the differences among camp settings are minute; yet, the abilities called forth for athletic games are considerably different than for cabin discussion meetings. What changed was not personnel but tactics and behavior patterns. The style of dominance expression, the specific behaviors that various settings elicited, and not who was dominant or subordinate was setting dependent. Thus, an alpha asserted himself or herself physically during athletic games, but during group discussions he or she was more prone to argue.

In answer to the question, "Are dominance and altruism stable characteristics of individuals or of the system?", Bernstein (1980) argues that dominance and altruism are dynamic rather than static; they are properties of the individual only within certain social contexts and thus not permanent characteristics of the individual. If "of the system," then individuals should vary in rank by setting or activity; but they did not in the present studies. Most likely there is a plurality of determinants, some tied to morphological and temperamental inheritance and others to socialization factors. This degree is probably flexible and defines a range of possibilities rather than a precise positional placement. The range depends on other factors, such as who else is present, and on characteristics of the setting. The reaction of the subordinate may be critical here. Due to previous interactions with another individual she or he may subordinate herself or himself. The subordinate may recognize physical (size, muscularity), behavioral (vigor, confidence), or social (kinship) characteristics that connote relative status (Bernstein, 1980).

If six alphas were placed together in a group, it is obvious that not all would be "most dominant"; if an omega adolescent were placed in a group of juvenile individuals two to three years younger, it is doubtful that she or he would reside at the bottom of the new dominance hierarchy. As with any trait, expression is context dependent. It would also be enlightening to observe the highly skilled athletic alphas in a music camp where the criterion of status might be music ability. Knowing these individuals, it is highly unlikely that such youth, accustomed to high status at camp, school, and neighborhood, would ever submit themselves to a situation with a risk of losing such favored status. Such "experiments" have not been undertaken, although they might be most instructive in describing the flexibility of adolescent behavior interactions.

Thus, I am in agreement with both Bernstein (1981) and his critics. On a molecular level dominance does not exist as a trait; the motor patterns involved in an act are dependent on the context and the outcome for a proper definition of "dominance" to apply. Moving to a higher level of analysis, however, I believe there is ample evidence in the research reported in this book to suggest a trait conception of dominance. That is, some adolescents consistently win or are recognized by peers as winners; others consistently lose, and this is a secret to few. Within hours of meeting each other these individual differences are apparent and form the initial and subsequent patterns of interaction.

My position is similar to the more general view that I take to Leeds (1984): The "dominance trait" is one of those "innumerable universals of human life" that has a biological basis that varies from one individual to another—and, perhaps, from some populations of individuals to others—but that depends for its specific exemplification in form, content, and timing by sociocultural factors such as physical setting (athletic field or church), social context (discussions or meditation), past and recent events that led up to its expression, who else is present (someone with high or low levels of the dominance trait), and how the culture allows one to express power (physical or verbal). Thus, dominance is both an individual trait and a relationship; I view the dominance trait as an orientation, a predisposition dependent on social conditions. Although Leeds is usually credited with being an anti-sociobiologist, his views are in line with many ethologists who assume a more biosocial perspective of human behavior than that usually credited to Wilson (1975).

The present findings are thus consistent with a trait conceptualization of dominance and altruism. The evidence suggests that trait theories of personality do not have to be discarded—only that we need to revise our methods of studying them. Although a trait approach to personality stresses the importance of individual predispositions in determining behavior, this should not imply that the contribution of situational or interactional factors should be overlooked. Rather, the trait approach suggests that the adolescent and what he or she brings to those situations are significant determinants as well (e.g., Costa & McCrae, 1980). The present investigation illustrates the power of an observational methodology for studying personality among adolescents. If psychologists wish to obtain meaningful information about human personality and behavior, it is important to observe individuals in the contexts in which they live.

10
Developing Perspective

In this final chapter I weave together the book's apparent disparate strands. In Chapter 1 position papers on the future research agenda for the study of adolescence were reviewed; they were found wanting because, "Predictive science begins with description" (Candland & Hoer, 1981; p. 436), and few of the agenda setters advocated such a back-to-the-basics approach. The first section of this chapter contrasts information gleaned from an ethological paradigm versus a standard psychological model.

My response to the proposed agendas was to offer a counter-proposal, one that argued for the necessity of descriptive, naturalistic research that affirmed rather than ignored or denied our species' phylogenetic unity with other animals, especially other primates. The second section of this chapter explores the merits of the naturalistic approach, from a methodological point of view; the third and fourth sections, from an empirical examination of group structure and of the extremeties of that structure, the alphas and the omegas.

Ethologists must, by virtue of a theoretical "trade agreement," speculate as to the evolutionary nature of their phenomenon. With some amount of "informed" soul-searching, I address the adaptive effects of a dominance system among the Camp Wancaooah groups of adolescent males and females. This ethological perspective of dominance incorporates both biological and social aspects of development as they affect individuals through the adolescent years. This approach is, I believe, both healthier and more accurate; its application to a contemporary development, the Men's Movement, is used as an example. These issues are further elaborated in this chapter before the book closes with a final look at the participant observer.

Comparing Ethological and Psychological Methodologies[1]

The match between what an individual reports on standardized paper-and-pencil tests, and how she or he behaves when interacting with others in natural settings should be a major issue in psychological research. But, the usual psychological procedure is to employ self-report measures to assess personality phenomena. Who but the individual, after all, is more qualified to make such judgments? Whether the individual actually behaves in the manner of the assessed personality characteristic is a blind spot for psychologists. Enter the ethologist who relies not so much on the verbal reports of subjects but on their behavior, as observed in naturalistic settings. The research reported here compares various psychological and ethological methods, including self-reports, behavioral observations, and peer rankings, to assess aspects of adolescent personality.

Two personality characteristics frequently assessed by both psychological and ethological researchers as independent and dependent variables are the themes of this book, dominance and altruism. Most self-report personality tests used by psychologists include dominance as a subscale or dimension (Butt & Fiske, 1968); as an interpersonal behavior dominance is frequently studied by ethologists (see reviews by Omark, Strayer, & Freedman, 1980; Savin-Williams & Freedman, 1977). Both psychologists and ethologists as well have taken an interest in altruism, as documented earlier in this book. In addition, a measure frequently employed by both human ethologists and psychologists, peer rankings, is used as a third method. The intent is to compare self-report, behavioral observation, and peer ranking methods of assessing individual personality, and thus to contrast the methodological approaches of human ethologists and psychologists.

Methods

The youth in this study were previously described as Study One participants in Chapter 8. Methods for data collection are reviewed in both Chapter 8 (altruism) and Chapter 9 (dominance). In addition, two self-report measures were given. The dominance subscale of the California Psychological Inventory (1964) (CPI) was administered to each group separately on the fifth day of camp. The subscale contains 46 items to which the respondent indicates agreement or disagreement ("I think I would enjoy having authority over other people.").

---

[1]This section is based on an earlier published paper (Savin-Williams, Small, & Zeldin, 1981).

A self-report measure of altruism, the Schwartz Ascription of Responsiblity Scale (1968), was adminstered to the 12 youth during the first week of camp. The Schwartz utilizes a five-point scale ranging from strong agreement to strong disagreement to measure an individual's tendency to ascribe to the self responsibility for the welfare of others ("I wouldn't feel that I had to do my part in a group project if everyone else was lazy.").

Results

Dominance. In each group the youth were given four rank order scores (Table 10.1) based on dyadic dominance, behavioral frequency of dominance, peer perceptions of dominance, and CPI dominance self-reports. Spearman rank order intercorrelations were computed among these four scores (Table 10.2). The two behavioral scores were significantly intercorrelated, and each was significantly related to peer perceptions of dominance. These three, however, were not significantly correlated with the CPI subscale of dominance completed by each individual.

Altruism. Within each group the adolescents were assigned three rank order scores (Table 10.1): behavioral frequency of altruism, peer perceptions of altruism, and Schwartz scores. Spearman rank order intercorrelations were computed among these three scores (Table 10.2). Although the frequency of prosocial acts was significantly related to peer perceptions of helpfulness and the self-report responsibility scores (Schwartz),

TABLE 10.1. Rank Order Scores for Measures of Dominance and Altruism for Two Groups

	Dominance				Altruism		
	Dyad	Freq	Peer	CPI	Freq	Peer	Swtz
Group A							
Alda	1	2	1	1.5	1	1	2
Geoff	2	1	2	4	6	5	4
Mick	3	3	3.5	1.5	2	3	1
Sven	4	4	3.5	3	4	6	3
Kit	5	6	6	6	5	4	6
Matt	6	5	5	5	3	2	5
Group B							
Evert	1	1	1	4	1	2	2
Carr	2	4	2	3	3	1	4
Tim	3	2	3	2	5	6	5
Gill	4	5	6	6	6	5	6
Orville	5	3	4	5	4	4	3
Dick	6	6	5	1	2	3	1

TABLE 10.2. Spearman Rank Order Intercorrelations and Chi-Squares for Combining Probabilities from Independent Samples for Dominance and Altruism

	Group A			Group B			Combined
	r	p	χ^a	r	p	χ^a	χ^a
Dominance							
Dyad–Freq	.89	.02	7.30	.71	.07	5.15	12.45*
Dyad–Peer	.93	.01	8.27	.83	.03	6.65	14.92**
Dyad–CPI	.76	.05	5.76	−.14	.59	1.04	6.80
Freq–Peer	.93	.01	8.27	.77	.05	5.76	14.03**
Freq–CPI	.65	.10	4.51	−.14	.59	1.04	5.55
Peer–CPI	.76	.05	5.76	.20	.37	1.96	7.72
Altruism							
Freq–Peer	.77	.05	5.78	.77	.05	5.78	11.56*
Freq–Swtz	.66	.09	4.69	.89	.02	7.30	11.99*
Peer–Swtz	.20	.37	1.96	.54	.15	3.72	5.68

[a]See Gordon, Loveland, and Cureton, 1952
*$p < .05^2$
**$p < .01$

the peer perception and Schwartz scores were not significantly correlated with each other.

Methodological Perspectives on Research

The nonbehavioral orientation and the reliance on paper-and-pencil measures of psychologists disturb a number of researchers other than ethologists. For example, Shweder (1975), in a reanalysis of four classic psychological studies, compared results from various personality measures (relationship of conceptual schemes, rated behavior, interpersonal ratings by group members and external observers, and self-reports on three personality inventories) to actual behavior. His failure to discover any significant relationship of the personality measures with the behavioral reports led him to question the concept of personality:

The challenge held out to personality psychology by this paper is to empirically support with observational data the applicability of the concept "personality" in its "individual difference" sense. The analyses suggest it is considerably less relevant for accounts of behavior than is generally supposed although the possibility that it is pertinent in certain restriced domains (e.g., with regard to hereditable characteristics such as activity level), should not be dismissed. (p. 480)

Although too frequently research infers an individual's normative behavior from self-report inventories or single observations in laboratory settings, there is a growing consensus that personality assessment must involve a direct measurement of behavior in the settings in which it naturally occurs:

The future of personality measurement will be brighter if we can move beyond our favorite pencil-and-paper and laboratory measures to include direct observation as well as unobtrusive nonreactive measures to study lives where they are really lived and not merely where the researcher finds it convenient to look at them. (Mischel, 1977; p. 248)

The rationale for applying direct measurement methods (e.g., observing naturally occurring behavior) is based on a number of considerations.

Self-Reports

The findings reported in this book on dominance and altruism give divergent views on the relationship between how a male adolescent says he behaves, and how he actually behaves when observed in naturalistic settings. How dominant an adolescent said he was on a personality inventory was not predictive of his behaviorally based or peer assessed dominance status. By contrast, how frequently he helped others in his group was significantly related to his self-reported level of social and personal responsibility; peer perceptions were related to behavioral altruism, but not self-report altruism. Two possible explanations for these discrepant results come to mind. First, due to the nature of early adolescence, it may be extremely difficult for boys to accurately report an issue of such psychological centrality as peer dominance status.

From a psychological and an ethological perspective, adolescence is generally portrayed as a time of heightened concern with status relations among peers. As the pubescent individual moves from the parental unit to the more external world, the peer group frequently becomes the forum of transition and high peer status may have important consequences in both the psychological (self-esteem, popularity, careers) and ethological (gene pool distribution, propagation of the species, access to scarce resources) realms. Although the adolescent boys at Camp Wancaooah tended to overrank themselves on all dimensions measured, they were most egocentric on the peer status items, dominance and popularity.

Because peer dominance status is of such psychological and ethological importance to the individual, it may be difficult for an adolescent to accurately self-report his dominance standing in the peer group, especially if that status is less than that desired by the individual. There is little evidence, however, that altruism is of such central psychological concern during the early adolescent years. Erikson (1959) proposes that it is during later stages of the life course when issues of personal and social responsibility and concern reach their normative peak. Consequently, early adolescents may be more willing and capable to adequately reflect on their prosocial behavior; thus, these two methods of assessing altruism match.

A second explanation for the present findings, congruent with the interests of interactional psychologists (Endler & Magnusson, 1976; Magnusson & Endler, 1977), stems from differences in the role that situational factors play in the expression of dominance and altruism. From this perspective both the characteristics of a situation (physical setting, activity, others present) as well as predispositions (both genetic and deeply ingrained cultural) that an individual brings to the situation are crucial in determining behavior.

As discussed in Chapter 9, because dominance behavior is considerably more dependent on interpersonal characteristics of the situation than is altruism, in order to accurately predict dominance behavior, one needs to know not only the degree of the "dominance trait" that an individual brings with him to a situation, but also the characteristics of the other individuals present (Bernstein, 1981; Gottman & Ringland, 1981). Thus, an individual is most likely to exhibit a high degree of dominance when there is both a strong dominance disposition and the situational characteristics are conducive to its expression (i.e., individuals are present who will respond submissively to the actor). By contrast, the performance of altruistic behavior is less dependent on interpersonal factors. In the present study altruistic behavior was performed by an actor for the benefit of another individual who did not, however, necessarily have to be in need of assistance or aid (e.g., an individual is given candy), be receptive to being helped, or even involved in the interactions (e.g., one individual making hot chocolate for the group).

Therefore, a self-report measure may be unable to predict dominance behavior due to its inability to provide information concerning characteristics of both the person and the situation; altruism, however, is less dependent on the interpersonal characteristics of the situation. Consequently, a self-report measure is able to adequately predict a person's altruistic tendencies given information concerning only the target individual.

Naturalistic Observations

Sommer (1977) noted that, "Psychology entered the laboratory almost a century ago and has not yet recovered from the experience". (p. 1) We know considerably more about the laboratory rat in a maze than about the wild rat in his or her natural habitat. "We have developed a science of pyschology based largely on behavior in the laboratory and have hedged on the issue of generalization". (Sommer, 1977; p. 7) Somehow studying animals—including humans—in cages has come to be identified as "real psychology." And we have even failed to study "normal caged human behavior." Rather than studying inmates locked in isolation, psychologists pay volunteers to submit themselves to sensory isolation experiments under antiseptic conditions to explore the effects of solitary confinement (Sommer, 1977). Psychology's chosen problems and methods have become increasingly "esoteric and hermetic."

A number of researchers in personality and socialization (Bronfenbrenner, 1979; Buss & Craik, 1980; Epstein, 1980; Mischel, 1977) have proposed that the most adequate methodological solution to many of the problems noted above resides in employing the kinds of direct measurement procedures most frequently used by ethologists:

One evident next step in this line of research calls for field studies, entailing prototypicality ratings of acts observed *in situ*. ... Such naturalistic field studies, providing fuller elaboration and documentation of dispositional concepts, are urgently needed in personality research. (Buss & Craik, 1980; p. 390)

This research approach is considerably more formidible than the relatively easy procedures of the one-shot self-reports used by many personality researchers. One advantage of an ethological methodology is that it encourages an assessment of the immediate situation and its multi-determinants (including the behavior of both the initiator and the recipient). By contrast, most psychological methodologies such as self-report inventories traditionally place the emphasis on the individual, and only minimally consider the characteristics of the situation. Ethology is thus in part congruent with the emergence of interactional approaches to personality while still maintaining its commitment to cross-age, cross-cultural, and cross-species comparisons.

Employing such a research strategy is not, however, without its disadvantages. In contrast to self-report measures and single occasion laboratory experiments, collecting data *in situ* carries a high cost of time and the sample size is usually small, thus limiting the power of statistical tests and generalizations to other populations. Other potential problems include the observer systematically affecting that which he or she is or is not observing (e.g., Webb, Campbell, Schwartz & Sechrest, 1966) and inherent biases in observers that may affect the reliability of their observations (e.g., Cantor & Mischel, 1977).

The present findings suggest that naturalistic observation is not as difficult as it might appear to be. For example, differences between individuals observed after only four days were significantly similar to differences observed two to four weeks later; thus, even brief periods of intensive observation may yield potent data. In addition, not only do the high correlations between peer perceptions and observed behavior tend to dispel the possibility of observer bias, they also suggest that even among untrained observers, a high degree of reliability can be obtained.

I believe that the benefits of an observation methodology outweigh the costs. To gain a better understanding of adolescent behavior, it is imperative to observe individuals in naturalistic settings. Regardless of the disadvantages that an observational approach might possess, with an increasing awareness of the complexity of behavior and the limitations of traditional methods of assessment, other ways of investigating behavior and personality must be found.

The decision to employ naturalistic research methods, however, depends on the question asked. For example, if the question concerns individual or a group of individuals, then an experimental method interacts, then a naturalistic approach may be appropriate. If the issue, however, is to delineate whether a specific event has a certain effect on an individual or a group of individuals, then an expermental method including relevant controls may be more useful (McCall, 1977). Indeed, it may be the combination of naturalistic and experimental methods that can best contribute to our understanding of human development, but only if our knowledge of the normative occurrence of behavior is adequate for the persons or phenomena under study to warrant experimental methods. Sommer (1977; p. 7) notes "... if we want to generalize from lab to life, we are going to have to learn more about life too." As I argued in Chapter 1, adolescents have not yet been brought to life and the study of adolescence has not yet reached this level of sophistication.

Ecological Validity

Another methodological consideration concerns the issue of ecological validity, defined by Bronfenbrenner (1979, p. 29) as, "The extent to which the environment experienced by the subjects in a scientific investigation has the properties it is supposed or assumed to have by the investigator." It is often difficult for staged settings to achieve ecological validity. Not only is there a possibility of a subject reacting to the strangeness of the laboratory setting (Orne, 1973), but it is also difficult to create a range of situations that is representative of an individual's normative environment. For example, Benson and his colleagues (1980) suggested that prosocial behavior, studied as a single isolated event in the laboratory where the experimenter defines the helping situation, is highly influenced by situational factors. They posit, however, that normative prosocial behavior that occurs outside of the laboratory, where the benefactor is left to his or her own resources and actively seeks out the helping event, tends to be more influenced by intrapersonal factors such as personality, values, and, I would add, biological predisposition. Thus, ecological validity is best obtained through naturalistic research methods.

Unless the research question concerns an individual's self-perception, the direct observation of behavior also has greater face validity than self-report measures because it is based on how an individual actually behaves in specific situations. Self-reports, on the other hand, are based on judgments of how one thinks he or she has acted, would act, or should act in a particular setting. Thus, although self-report measures are easy to administer, direct observation of behavior frequently has more utility and is, I believe, more valid.

Multiple Forms

Using a variety of forms for a construct encourages cross-species and cross-cultural comparisons. For example, supplanting others, gaining access to priorities, displaying threat gestures, and receiving attention from others are behaviors that define dominance in both human and nonhuman primate adolescents. In the early adolescent groups, however, the primary mode of expressing status was verbal, roughly 70%, thus highlighting the symbolic, linguistic skills of humans. Any definition of dominance or altruism that is applicable to only one species or to a limited range of behavior, such as aggression or sharing, is doomed to obsolescence as a narrow and ungeneralizable tool. It is imperative to explicitly define and to use a multidimensional approach to the study of behaviors. At least this is an ethological view of the situation.

Group Structure

Based on the observation methodology presented in this book, a number of conclusions can be proposed concerning adolescent behavior. In dyadic encounters with other same-sex, same-age peers, adolescents behave in a fashion that can be summarized on a group level as either a dominance hierarchy or a cohesive dyarchy. For adolescent males ages 10 through 17 years a stable and ordered, but not invariant group structure can be assessed not only through observations of interpersonal behavior, but also through the verbal reports of group members. For adolescent females I am less sure about the nature of the group structure, although it is clear that a hierarchical structure exists. The incorporation of new group members or the exchange of cabin counselors for a day does little to disrupt the dyadic behavior patterns.

A standard, acceptable means for constructing a group hierarchy from the behaviors observed is needed (Strayer, 1980). Several methods have been used, making cross-study comparisons difficult. For example, group members have been arranged on the basis of (1) the percentage of dyadic interactions in which one is the dominant member, (2) the frequency of dominance acts, (3) the number of group members dominated, and (4) sociometric rankings of informed others, independent sources, and/or the group participants.

There are problems with these methods. Nonhuman primate studies indicate that the frequency with which an animal enters into dominance interactions is not always related to his or her position in the group hierarchy. This has also been noted for humans (Pitcairn & Strayer, 1984):

Exclusive attention to rates of initiation of aggression, or elicited submission, without reference to the dyadic context of such activities, may provide a meaningful measure of individual differences, but such differences can be totally unrelated to social roles within the group dominance structure. (p. 371)

The most active animal is often a beta or a middle ranked individual who may be attempting to defend a position or to advance in the hierarchy (Southwick, 1972). This was often the case with the early adolescents at Camp Wancaooah. The antagonistic or bully camper was frequently most involved in cabin dominance encounters, but she or he was rarely the most dominant individual in the group.

Proportion of total acts in which one is dominant may also result in a biased hierarchical arrangement. A group member may have her or his dominance success percentage "padded" by constantly dominating low ranking group members, a higher percentage than if interactions were primarily with those closest to one's own rank.

The method emphasized here to construct a group structure was inspired by Goodall's (1968) point that a population per se does not develop a hierarchy—it is only established in interindividual relations that may have meaning for the total group—and by Tinbergen's (1953) examination of social organization at the level of interactions between two individuals. It was also considered important not to isolate the dyads from the ongoing naturalistic social situation, as might be done in contrived laboratory studies. Using these assumptions Weisfeld and Weisfeld (1984) also found dyadic analysis of dominance behaviors among adolescent boys playing volleyball to be more useful than a mere frequency count of dominance interactions.

Because they use pre-existing groups, previous studies on dominance are seldom informative in regard to the process by which a dominance hierarchy is formed and maintained over time. Although it is difficult to determine the exact point in the life of an ongoing group that relative dominance status is recognized by group members, in new groups "end anchoring," the identification of extreme stimuli in a series and the judgment of others relative to those extremes (Sherif & Sherif, 1964), occurs within hours of meeting in both male and female groups. Opening day dyadic interactions in the present studies frequently set a five week pattern. The "end anchors," the alphas and the omegas, were most consistently recognized among both early and late adolescents. Not addressed—and yet potentially most informative—is the disintegration of a group's life.

In the camp studies the group structure became more stable over time, with most dyadic relationships becoming firmly entrenched. The contested or flexible dyadic relationships were predictable, resulting in occasional shifts in relative status occurring between adjacently ranked group members (one up, one down). This basic hierarchical stability may extend over a long period of time.

Alphas and Omegas

Nonhuman primate research has seldom undertaken the task of predicting the group dominance structure by reference to individual characteristics of all group members. Research on humans has occasionally attempted such procedures, but with little success. Few physical, behavioral, or social measures (e.g., age, body size, aggression, sociability, experience, popularity) consistently or significantly predict the dominance status of all group members (Savin-Williams & Freedman, 1977), for reasons noted by Bernstein (1981) in Chapter 2 (e.g., one's rank depends on who else is in the group).

The nonhuman primate literature suggests that a more productive technique than relating the entire rank order to some dimension is to examine the characteristics of individuals at the extreme points of the hierarchy. Monkey and ape adolescent alpha males tend to be morphologically larger and physically stronger than their peers. On the other hand, "social graces" with a "pleasing personality" are as important as physical size and strength in many primate species for attaining a prominent position in the group. An alpha is the center of attention, a focal animal for unification of the group. Although not always the leader in trail progressions, a top ranked individual leads in the sense of initiating and directing group movement. Such an individual defends the group against both internal and external sources of disturbances (Savin-Williams, in press). Dominant chimpanzees are not only stronger but also more highly motivated, coordinated, and "ingenious" than are subordinates (Goodall, 1968).

With increasing frequency, ethologists, social psychologists, and political scientists have renewed their attempts to predict interpersonal dominance and submission status on the basis of physical, nonverbal features (reviewed in Ellyson & Dovidio, 1985). Studies focusing on human children and adolescents indicate that the most dominant individual is generally older, taller, heavier, tougher, and healthier and is more popular, athletic, daring, and attractive then other group members. On the other hand, low ranking children are timid, asocial, passive or hostile, unpopular, "different," and cold (personality) (Savin-Williams & Freedman, 1977).

Both male and female alpha ranked young adolescents in the current study were similar in style of dominance expression and in several physical and social traits. Leaders in the cabin group, alphas were more indirect than most cabinmates when asserting their power and authority, which were usually expressed through verbal directives. During cabin discussions their suggestions and ideas were frequently adhered to by others. As camp progressed alphas became less involved in intragroup dominance interactions than they were previously during the first weeks of camp. Cabinmates frequently recognized the leader's superior status, and they remembered years later when asked to recount the cabin hierarchy. Almost all remembered that alpha was alpha.

Alphas were not necessarily early maturers, but in relation to agemates they were pubertally mature, tall and heavy, and slightly old. Most were also judged to be physically attractive, intelligent, and athletic. They were liked by the counselors and by their peers. In the all-camp data, alpha males at all ages (10 to 15 years) were characterized by peers and counselors as athletic, pubertally mature, popular, and non-problem campers. In short, they were a delight to have in the group, relieving the cabin counselor of many leadership responsibilities.

Alphas were portrayed by peers as self-confident, physically and socially appropriate, "cool," mature, and popular; omega ranked young adolescents were viewed as insecure, physically and socially clumsy, "embarrassing," and too talkative and friendly. As a group only several months younger than the leaders, they averaged two years less pubertally mature. The late maturing males were two inches shorter and 20 pounds lighter than the top ranked individuals. In most cases they were the worst athlete in the cabin, and they suffered as a result.

These "submissive followers" or "compliant clingers" frequently called attention to their subordinate position by recognizing the dominance status of cabinmates. They appeared to be extremely vulnerable adolescents, monitoring surroundings as if they expected to be ridiculed, which was an almost universal reaction to them, or to gauge appropriate behavior. When it occurred, dominance over cabinmates was usually achieved through verbal arguments and overt forms of behavior.

Effects of a Dominance System

Ethologists assume that a systematic group structure, whether patterned as a dominance hierarchy or as a cohesive dyarchy, develops and is maintained because individuals and/or the group benefit(s) from such a structure. Alexander (1974) concluded that groups "form and persist" because all members gain genetically. Weisfeld and Linkey (1985) supported their view that "success striving" or dominance is an evolved characteristic in humans by documenting its universality in human cultures and its maturational, genetic pattern within an individual. In addition, the neural mediation and phylogenetic continuity, through parallel displays and emotional signals, of dominance behavior support its evolved basis.

Given the ethological studies conducted to date, however, the evolutionary advantage of a particular status position is a matter of speculation. It is possible, however, to demonstrate more proximate, "personal benefits" that an individual derives from a dominance position. For example, the high ranking early adolescents at camp frequently ate the biggest piece of cake at mealtimes, sat where they wanted to during discussions, and slept in the preferred sleeping sites during campouts (near the fire)—all "scarce resources" at camp. These are not unlike the benefits other primate adolescents gain from high status. Subadult male langurs base accessibility to food, right of way, and tree position on relative dominance rank (Yoshiba, 1968). It is difficult empirically, however, to distinguish prerogatives of rank from determinants and expressions of rank:

> It seems reasonable to suppose that volleyball ability determined rank in this setting, and that access to the ball and the chance to evaluate others constituted prerogatives. However, evaluating others may also have raised a S's rank, by acting as either a bluff or a sign of high rank. A single behavior might constitute a determinant, a prerogative, and an expression of rank simultaneously. (Weisfeld & Weisfeld, 1984; p. 97)

Perhaps the most salient benefit from high status is internal. Levi-Strauss (1951) noted that even in cultures where being a leader may result in personal loss or death, some individuals strive for the position because of its intrinsic reward, an enhanced self-esteem. Chance (1967) suggested that the most dominant male individual is the focus of attention within the group. Others imitate him, seek his support, and allow him to innovate without inhibition from other group members (McGrew, 1972). In nonhuman primates Washburn and Hamburg (1968) noted that "being dominant appears to be its own reward—to be highly satisfying and to be sought, regardless of whether it is accompanied by advantage in food, sex, or grooming" (p. 473). Itani (1961) suggested renaming the power hierarchy, "prestige" hierarchy. McGuinness (1984) referred to this as a "desire to be assertive." Alpha nonhuman primates appear to their human observers to be "confident" animals. In support of this, there was a highly significant relationship between dominance and self-esteem among the late adolescent females. Of those boys who returned to Camp Wancaooah for another summer, former beta males were the most numerous, perhaps to achieve, with the benefit of another summer at camp, the alpha position.

The most dominant adolescents were not only perceived by peers as possessing ideal leadership traits, but they also acted as if they were the leaders. A leader might not necessarily suggest the most ideas, but the ones she or he wanted were readily perceived by cabinmates as acceptable. Frequently, low status members did not express their opinion or vote until higher ranking individuals made their desires and judgments known. Because leadership was behaviorally defined as dominance over the group as a whole (in terms of the group doing what was wanted), it is not surprising that leadership correlated so highly (average of .87) with a rank order based on the sum of group individuals significantly dominated in pair-wise interactions.

Not all, however, strive to be alpha; but there is little speculation as to the personal benefits of a subordinate rank. Sherif and Sherif (1964) suggested that all group members want to feel a sense of belonging and that they are acceptable to the peer group. To achieve this security some group members are willing to submit. Alexander (1974) is more explicit:

The subordinate also gains by his behavior: like the dominant he is informed by the interactions of the hierarchy when and how to display aggression, and when and how to withhold and appease and withdraw, so as to stay alive and remain in the group and be at least potentially reproductive for the longest period. (p. 330)

Many of the subordinate adolescents at Camp Wancaooah appeared to identify with the group's success and to accept their status as a way of life. They avoided, with a passion, making decisions and being responsible for others. Deciding which way to travel on a strange path or which of several foods to take on a campout was not an enjoyable or sought after task for some adolescents. Perhaps the maxim "everyone cannot be a leader" should be altered to include the words, "nor wants to be." Although ranked last, omega adolescents had a more preferred position than not having any place in the group. One sensed that during the normal year omegas were loners or not really part of a peer group. They were likely to return to Camp Wancaooah the next summer, perhaps because there was an increased likelihood of upward mobility with succeeding years at camp, or because they wanted the sense of belonging which was readily available at camp.

In other primate groups it has been suggested that the advantages of a dominance hierarchy are to alleviate the damaging aspects of aggression without decreasing its survival value (defense of self and group, predator protection, altruism, delineation of habitat) and to add stability and expectancy to social living (Eibl-Eibesfeldt, 1975). According to a recent conference (McGuinness, 1984), knowledge of dominance status within the group reduces stress and ambiguity, diminishes aggression, and provides a harmonious environment.

Because of their group status, particular individuals have specialized obligations and roles to perform, expected of them by other group members. Failure to carry out these duties implies loss of the prestige that has been bestowed by the group (Thrasher, 1927). From a more egotistical point of view Alexander (1974, p. 327) notes: "Whenever individuals derive benefits from group functions they may be expected to carry out activities that maintain the group, and thereby serve their own interests as well."

High ranking human adolescents played a crucial, instrumental role within the camp group. Arguments during athletic games were reduced to a minimum when the alpha individual, by assessing everyone's athletic skills, told each where to play and for how long. Few objected to this authoritarianism, even those low ranking cabinmates who frequently had to play undesirable (right field, defensive back) positions. The most dominant individuals initiated and determined group movement; they also made the important decisions within the cabin group, such as deciding the theme of the cabin flag or where to camp on the beach. The subordinates' role was to do the necessary work for the implementation and completion of tasks, and to follow.

As previously discussed, the female pattern added another dimension by differentiating the instrumental and expressive dominance status positions within the group. The top ranked expressive girl concerned herself with the more intrapersonal and interpersonal issues within the group. When intermeshing properly, the net effect of their behavior and the behavior of subordinates was the stabilization of interpersonal relations and an enhanced group performance.

The level of serious fights in the cabin groups studied was extremely low, 1% of the over 7000 dominance encounters observed among the early adolescents, and lower in the older adolescent groups. In the male adolescent groups the number of recorded dominance encounters dropped precipitously during camp; even though the level of antagonistic behavior tended to increase in female adolescent groups, behavior became more indirect in form as camp progressed. Thus, with stabilization of the group structure antagonistic behavior became either less frequent or less overt.

The group benefits by having dominant individuals within the group: Decisions are made, activities are organized, intragroup friction is avoided or reduced, and intragroup relationships are negotiated. With assigned or assumed group roles and obligations given to particular group members, a cohesive and well-functioning group was the result, and interindividual behavior was regulated in such a way so as to reduce the level of intraspecific aggression, beneficial to individuals and to the survival of the group.

Observers of adolescent groups recognize the essential quality and importance of the natural dominance group structure that serves to reduce fighting and conflict and to encourage group living and cooperation:

The boys' worker must work *with* the natural forces and mechanisms in the gang rather than against them; his function is to lead and direct, rather than to impose something foreign from without. (Thrasher, 1927; p. 237)

A study of a lower class black Chicago neighborhood (Scheinfeld, 1973) revealed similar findings. In the adolescent hangout, a social network with clearly differentiated status positions was continuously reinforced. Individuals of lowest status were referred to as "reptiles" or as "pussys"—weakminded, used by others, dependent, no self-respect. They were held in contempt by the "regulars," the middle status individuals who formed the bulk of the peck order system, and by the "shonuf regulars," the elite of the hustlers. Much like higher socioeconomic alphas, these latter individuals were described by peers as "men"—have sense and "mother's wit" (an inner sense that tells one to take a particular direction) and are "nobody's fool." Most of all, a shonuf regular is "mellow"—an allright guy who is trustworthy, fair, generous, smart, informed, authentic, free, swift, and confident and who has a strong inner direction. Physical prowess is important in the sense of being able and ready to use violence if need be, an essential ingredient to gain and maintain peer respect in the black neighborhood. But, violence is also "anti-mellow" because it implies resorting to physical rather than mind force. The high status individual or elite group must prevent violence; otherwise, people are hurt, bringing the police.

In many respects the present study simply added numbers to the Chicago studies of Thrasher and Scheinfeld. Both were naturalistic observations of same-sex, young adolescent groups. Thrasher's "two-boy pals" is my dyad, the primary structure of the social organization; his natural social order based on disciplined sub- and super-ordination is my dominance hierarchy. We both found the group structure to be stable, yet plastic, and to function as a vehicle for social role clarification, aggression control, and perhaps, the development of identity (self-esteem). Qualities of the leader were also congruent: athletic, strong, big, experienced, intelligent, daring, convincing, firm, and self-confident—one who leads, directs, organizes, and inspires. Furthermore, the "styles of dominance and submission," that were developed independently of Thrasher's adolescent gang roles, are nearly identical with his leader, funny boy, show-off, goat, and sissy categories. Scheinfeld's work suggest that although there may be cross-cultural and cross-racial differences within the adolescent group, the similarity in the group structure, the individual characteristics necessary to achieve dominance, and the function of the social organization between his work and that reported here implies these may be universal phenomena.

Pubescence and Adolescence

In both nonhuman and human primates pubescence precipitates a major shift in the biosocial status of an individual. Physiologically, hormonal changes alter the biological substrate of drives, interests, emotions, and states of awareness, and, thus, one's threshold for behavioral sensitivity and reactivity in interpersonal encounters. Socially, now that the adolescent appears more sexually mature, others perceive these outward changes and react accordingly, with the concommitant effects on an adolescent's self-perception, and on his or her social behaviors. As an individual looks more like a man or a woman, others are more likely to expect adult-like behaviors, including appropriate dominance and altruistic behaviors.

With the new physical features accompanying pubescence, such as primary genitalia development and secondary sex character growth in hips, breast, chest, beard, and pubic hair, one's social status will likely be affected, thus illustrating the blend of the biological and the social. For example, an increase in testosterone level at pubescence initiates the male facial hair development that in turn, may be threatening to other males— thus enhancing one's dominance status. Or, one may view the upward testosterone level as partial causation of an increased sexual drive that motivates an individual to seek a sexual encounter which may also affect one's peer status.

The relative merits of biological and social explanations of behavior will probably never be settled for the satisfaction of either discipline. One recent study (Udry et al., 1985) reaches a level of biosocial sophistication that typifies what I believe will ultimately prevail. Serum hormone assays were performed on a population of 102 13-16 year old boys to assess their contribution to the sexual maturation and behavior of the sample. Their results indicate (1) that socially learned rules prescribe when to date, and what should be the progressive sequence of sexual behavior (from kissing to coitus) and (2) that a biologically based variable predicts the level of one's sexual motivation and sexual behavior. They concluded that " ... our data strongly suggest that the degree of involvement in these socially determined patterns of sexual behavior is heavily influenced by serum androgenic hormones ... (that) work directly through biologically based motivation and not through the social interpretation of the associated pubertal development." (Udry et al., 1985; p. 94)

This example illustrates the possible combinatorial power of the biological and social dimensions. Other disciplines have also noted this fact:

Our haste to seek out the one best explanation delays our better sense that the normal adolescent lives both in the inside and in the outside of his body, in rough correspondence to the depth of psychoanalysis and to the surface of social-learning ... The adolescent literally turns a new face and body to the world around him and, through his appearance to others, recognizes himself as one who approaches, for better or worse, the physical stature and psychosocial status of adulthood. (Peskin, 1973; p. 274)

The link between biological pubescence and social status was documented in the current studies; although pubertal maturation was one of the few variables that significantly correlated with dominance status during early adolescence, it was not so highly related when pubertal maturation is essentially completed during late adolescence.

The primary focus in these naturalistic studies was on early adolescence because it is during the age of pubescence, regardless of the primate species, when social competitive behavior increases and group bonding and allegiance are formulated for both males and females. The peer group may become influential as the adolescent consolidates his or her sense of self by comparison against the norms or standards of peer behaviors, attitudes, and values (Gilligan, 1982; Hartup, 1983; Kelley, 1952). Hence, the importance of dominance behavior (competitiveness) and hierarchical status (peer group status) in the adolescent peer group (group bonding and allegiance) becomes understandable. Erikson's (1959) notion of adolescence as a time of identity formation offers a psychological explanation for the awareness of, adherence to, and maintenance of the group. Because an essential ingredient in formulating and consolidating an identity is the discovery of one's place among one's peers, a dominance hierarchy or cohesive dyarchy that is relatively stable across time and activity, and that is clearly discernible to all aids the indentity process for all group members.

From an ethological perspective the end of pubescence is biological and social adulthood. Dominance behavior, thus, has a new importance during adolescence: The net outcome of one's dominance encounters with other group members may well determine one's relative adult status. The stability of dominance status over an extended period of time has been documented (Weisfeld, Omark, & Cronin, 1980; Weisfeld et al., in preparation). This status may once have had significance for one's relative genetic potential in both the number and the quality (potential to survive) of offspring produced. The outcome, at some point in the primates' evolutionary history, of such encounters may well have shaped what adolescents are today.

The position taken here is that when individuals freely interact, some are more likely than are others to rise to the top of a hierarchy, and others to fall to the bottom. This is also the position of McGuire (1974) who argues that in many primate groups some animals are compelled toward achieving a high dominance status. He outlines the role of genetic and environmental factors in his "idiosyncratic male hypothesis":

The hypothesis assumes that certain males are particularly assertive and aggressive by virtue of their genetic makeup. One essential element of this hypothesis, therefore, is genetic. Depending upon conditions of upbringing, such as mother's rank, n, social structure, etc., a certain amount of aggressiveness is more or less likely to manifest itself. But no conditions have been found which would suggest that continual intense aggressiveness, as seen in the fission process, is environmentally determined. Males that exhibit this continual intense aggressive behavior are called *idiosyncratic males*, i.e., their behavior does not appear to be the result of social conditions alone (although given conditions would theoretically enhance or suppress such behavior). (p. 124)

Other group members—whether for biochemical, morphological, temperamental, or socialization reasons—seem "satisfied" with low status.

Although it has not yet been discovered, the existence of an alpha "G" trait is not an unreasonable assumption. It is doubtful that the dominance G can be significantly suppressed, but it may be possible to alter the expression of dominance into behavioral patterns that are not destructive to the individual or to the group. This may be important for a youth worker who encounters a "bully" or "bitch" in the cabin group. Such youths may be more easily convinced by the adult to become less physically aggressive than to become less dominant.

Observers of human development seldom deny that biology influences developmental processes—who wants to be accused of being simpleminded?—but it is usually only acknowledged to exist while environmental, socialization processes receive the bulk of attention. For proof, examine most developmental psychology courses taught in colleges and universities in the United States; they recognize the importance of biology, but because most developmental psychologists are also *social* scientists, environmental influences on development receive greater airplay. In part this may be due to their perception that biology implies the status quo, determinism, and reactionary politics. This simplistic and wrong-headed view of biology is not limited to developmental psychologists (e.g., Lewontin, Rose, & Kamin, 1984).

In her conference summary, McGuinness (1984) emphasized that the resolution to this issue involves understanding the importance of the interplay between the two: A substrate for a biological predisposition does not imply the immutability of that disposition to environmental influences. Ethologists may be just as interested in what can be changed as what remains constant. But, to work for change, it is imperative to know the constants, the biological constraints of behavior or behavioral patterns. This view appears to be lost by many pro-environmental social scientists and their causes—for example, the Men's Movement.

Gentle Men and Gender

During the last decade a quiet, slowly evolving revolution has begun in the United States that has deep ramifications for a biological interpretation of human behavior, specifically gender behavior. It is the Men's Movement, briefly traced in Astrachan (1984). The Movement began in the 1970s with consciousness-raising groups for men concerned with (1) relationships with other men, (2) the changing role of women in their lives, and (3) the male gender role. The first National Conference on Men and Masculinity met in 1975; six years later a national group for men was organized. Newsletters (*Brothers, Men's Studies Newsletter*), journals (*Men's Journal, Changing Men*), local organizations and workshops (e.g., Ithaca Men's Network; the Ithaca Planned Parenthood's Conference on Men and Masculinity), and more than a few books (e.g., David & Brannon, 1976; Farrell, 1974; Pleck, 1981) followed.

The primary issues have been divorce and custody laws, gay rights, and feminism; but one issue has predominated most consistently: male gender and sex role stereotypes. The concern has been to broaden—some advocate change—the possibilities of sex role for men to include more traditional feminine characteristics such as gentleness, sensitivity, affection, and understanding. Boys, especially during adolescence, are taught to be competitive and dominating. According to Cooper Thompson (1985), what needs to be changed are the messages that boys receive of what they are to be if they are to be real men:

1. Be strong, self-confident, self-reliant, independent, physically strong, and in control;
2. Be tough, aggressive, competitive, daring, willing to fight, dominant;
3. Seek status, a prestigeous career, admiration and respect from others, a good salary; and
4. Avoid anything feminine because to be feminized is the worst that can happen to a male in the eyes of his peers and the world.

What should be taught to adolescent males is to accept their vulnerability, to ask for help and support, to express feelings, to be gentle and nurturant, to cooperate with others, to use non-violence to resolve conflict, to accept attitudes and behaviors labeled feminine as necessary for full human development, to love other males, and to value and support the strength of women (Thompson, 1985).

The difficulty of implementing these tasks will baffle or surprise few, primarily because to be successful the Movement would need to change the very nature of Western culture, if not the distribution of genetic materials between the sexes in her citizens. These themes are prevalent ones, and are directly tied to the issue of the extent to which these negative characteristics of male sex role stereotypes are built into the genetic nature of being a male. If innate, then the possibility of complete change is annihilated, or certainly made difficult.

A popular view is that of Pleck (1981) who argues against the "prevalent" masculine sex role identity (MSRI) position of Western culture. The MSRI assumes "an *innate* psychological need for sex-typed traits" (p. 134, emphasis added). On the other hand, Pleck argues that sex-typed traits are the result of social approval and situational adaptation; his self-role discrepancy theory states, "Individuals suffer negative consequences when they fail to live up to sex roles" (p. 134). Sex role behavior is not innate, but is the result of socialization pressures to conform to (maladaptive and dysfunctional) sex role stereotypes and norms. He critiques the biological argument for the innate basis of the well-documented finding that males are more aggressive than females. His "review" of the literature is patently dated (nothing within seven years of the publication of his book, although other cited publications are as recent as his book's publication date) and highly selective. In each section of the appendix Pleck searches for anything less than absolute certainty in the biological argument for an innate aggressive predisposition; if found, then he dismisses the entire biological explanation.

Pleck's views, expressed in his writings and his position as one of the founders of the Men's Movement and the National Organization for Changing Men, are extremely influential. If aggression, dominance, toughness, assertiveness, and other "masculine" traits are inborn, he argues, then there is little hope for changing men; the Men's Movement is pointless and useless. A recent editorial in *Changing Men* (November 14, 1985) stated, "We identify ourselves as men who are *consciously* moving away from the strait jacket of male sex role stereotypes" (emphasis added). The Movement would have better appreciated the research reported in this book if dominance status had proven to be temporally unstable and contexually dependent—a different leader emerging for every time and place under the sun.

But, this is not the story the adolescents told in their questionnaires or revealed in their behavior. Rather, there was strong evidence for a dominance trait that remained stable over time and setting—and that was differentially distributed within the adolescent population. There is in the research reported in this book, however, good news for the Men's Movement.

First, if allowed to function with minimal interference from adult authority, male toughness was seldom expressed violently or physically. The dominance hierarchy appeared to serve a debilitating influence on aggression—severely limiting or suppressing its expression in ways other than in verbal or non-physical means (also see the evidence on this issue presented in McGuinness, in press).

Second, the most physically and verbally aggressive individuals were rarely the most dominant youth in the group, for either sex. Such individuals wielded little influence or power. The most dominant youth were more similar to a peer or maternal leader, expressing their influence through indirect, non-physical behavior. Unlike the bullies and antagonists, these youth were well liked by peers and adults alike.

Finally, and, perhaps, this will only please some of the pro-feminist male advocates, adolescent girls also expressed the "masculine" characteristics of toughness and assertiveness. Some girls consistently assumed precedence over other girls. Thus, dominance as a trait is not limited to males. Some adolescent girls were just as tough as some adolescent boys although as a group, females were more likely to be subtle and verbal in their dominance interactions—but dominant, nevertheless.

The Participant Observer

Three issues pertinent to observational methodology are here considered: my male bias in observing and discussing the construct of dominance; the role of the adult authority during participant observations; and the need for more social scientists who will also be observers of human behavior.

Science is seldom neutral, and neither is the observer of human behavior. Gilligan (1982) noted that the position of the observer alters what is seen, conceptually and, I would add, based on the recent realization of structural differences in the brain between the sexes (Lacoste-Utamsing & Holloway, 1982), perceptually. The male bias in both what is observed, and how theoretical sense is made of it, has been articulated by Hrdy (1981) in her book *The Woman That Never Evolved.* In developmental psychology male life is frequently presented as the norm and the female's life is considered deviant (Gilligan, 1982).

This male bias is most apparent in this book by my attempt to interpret dominance interactions among early adolescent females in terms of a dominance hierarchical construct. Clearly, human adolescent females engage in dominance encounters—the eight indices are sufficiently unisex—but, they do not verbally nor behaviorally view such interactions as constituting a linear status arrangement. The peer dominance rankings probably made little sense to them—and, indeed, in one-half of the female cabin groups members did not agree among themselves on the rank order, and in only one instance did this composite agree with the behavioral data. Paikoff's cohesive dyarchy would appear to be a more accurate assessment of female group structure, at least among older adolescents.

Other problems with participant observers have been described by Fine and Glassner (1979). One is the adult's visibility:

Like the white researcher in black society, the male researcher studying women (or vice versa), or the ethologist observing a distant tribal culture, there is no way in which the adult participant observer who attempts to understand a children's culture can pass unnoticed as a member of that group. . . . Due to age segregation in American society (Conger, 1971), it is unexpected for an adult to "hang out" with children's groups; the only legitimate adult-child interaction outside the research situation is based upon the authority of the adult. This authority structure is difficult or impossible to eliminate completely, and several problems are particular to participant observation research with children for that reason. (p. 153)

The observers in the studies reported here assumed as in Barker and Wright's (1955) classic investigation, that the presence of the participant observer was quickly accepted by the youth as one aspect of the natural environment. Owing to the nature of the study, the age group under investigation, and the premium placed on observing naturally occurring behavior, the use of videotape or film was considered both intrusive and impractical.

We knew we were not invisible and there were instances when that was altogether too apparent (see Chapters 4 and 5). It is my belief that too frequently adult authority intervenes where either it is not needed or is counterproductive. For example, with delinquent boys Polsky (1962) noted that many professional staffs have a seemingly vested interest in changing the values and personality of individual boys. But the cottage peer social organizations subvert their efforts. Esser (1973) believes it is important that youth workers realize that aggressive behavior of adolescent boys is "a basic form of organization based on threat, force, and intimidation, as this exists in any animal society" (p. 144). It is natural, to be expected, cannot be eliminated, and is useful for group and interpersonal cohesiveness—and it need not be, nor is it seldom ever, physical aggression that is used to maintain order.

Second week interactions in Cabin Two illustrate this point. Gene, a bully, was constantly ridiculing Omar, rhyming Omar's last name with a word that cannot be printed in nice books. Others in the cabin asked Gene to cool it, but he persisted. As the authority, I knew I could stop the name calling, but only in my presence. I hoped that the group members would work out a solution that resolved this dilemma; but I said nothing, waiting for the inevitable moment. On a campout Gene, perhaps invigorated by the beautiful morning, was especially intense in his anti-Omar remarks. Suddenly, Omar broke, pinning Gene with a flurry of screams, wildly flaying arms, and a tackle. Gene, the bully, was so overwhelmed by the wimpy Omar, and so totally embarrassed that he never again repeated the name. In my talk with Omar immediately following this episode, it was apparent, through his tears, that he was proud that for the first time in his life he had stood up to someone. Although Omar was to remain the omega, he had a new sense of self-confidence and peer respect that would not have evolved with a meddling authority act on the part of his counselor.

There are times of course when an adult authority has the ethical and legal responsibility to intervene. An adult's power differential role can be deemphasized, but it can never vanish, loosened but never—and should never—be eliminated. My point is only that adults too seldom trust the behavioral wisdom of youth. They are quite capable of a high level of self-regulation and jurisprudence (Fine & Glassner, 1979).

It is difficult to teach an aspiring observer of adolescents more than specific observational skills. But, this is rarely offered or encouraged in departments of psychology; one must do more than simply read about observational methodology; one must also be supervised in field observations and recording skills:

We have to give students specific skills for handling the richness, complexity and flow of ongoing behavior—courses in content analysis, behavioral mapping, observational methods, archival measurement and photography. (Sommer, 1977; p. 7)

Perhaps many of us, inherently, have observational skills, but they are atrophied through disuse and discouragement by former schooling (Sommer, 1977). The inquiring mind and the ability to ask questions of relevance and depth are the starting points. Some of the most successful observers have been individuals who are supportive, sympathetic, and approving of youth, and who have a sense of who they are. Adolescents can easily spot those who attempt to be someone other than who they are, that is, those who connote a false sense of being "with it" (Fine & Glassner, 1979; Hollingshead, 1975; Sherif & Sherif, 1953).

If we were to heed Tinbergen's call to bring psychology back to its roots, its descriptive phase, there would be a great demand for the participant observer:

It seems to me that one of the lessons we can draw from Lorenz's work is that our science will always need naturalists and observers as well as experimenters; we must, by a balanced development of our science, make sure that we attract the greatest possible variety of talent, and certainly not discourage the man with a gift for observation. Instead, we should attract such men, for they are rare; we must encourage them to develop their gifts of observation, and help them ask relevant questions with respect to what they have seen. (Tinbergen, 1963; p. 413)

It is my hope that this book will contribute to bringing out the closeted participant observer, to make the trade respectable once again. If not, our understanding of human development will be distorted and incomplete.

Appendix A: Early Adolescents

TABLE A-1. Summary of Group Dominance Hierarchies for the Entire Camp Session (%)[a]

Male Groups

Group 1	Alan	Bobby	Gary	Don	Ed	Oscar	Total
Alan	—	66	79	81	88	85	76
Bobby		—	76	86	86	88	63
Gary			—	86	62	92	47
Don				—	48	53	33
Ed				52	—	49	32
Oscar				47	51	—	29

Group 2	Ara	Bjorn	Gene	Doug	Ernie	Omar	Total
Ara	—	67	94	83	100	80	79
Bjorn		—	80	63	91	90	65
Gene			—	65	71	67	46
Doug				—	74	90	45
Ernie					—	58	24
Omar					42	—	21

Group 3	Alex	Guy	Eric	Orville			Total
Alex	—	86	89	97			91
Guy		—	41	65			46
Eric		59	—	57			29
Orville		43	—				29

Group 4	Andy	Gar	Delvin	Otto			Total
Andy	—	71	75	69			71
Gar		—	55	60			49
Delvin		45	—	53			44
Otto			47	—			40

Female Groups

Group 5	Amy	Betty	Gilda	Donna	Olivia	Total
Amy	—	65	64	72	87	73
Betty		—	64	75	92	67
Gilda			—	68	91	57
Donna				—	88	42
Olivia					—	10

Group 6	Ann	Becky	Gloria	Dottie	Opal	Total
Ann	—	62	58	86	90	71
Becky		—	57	80	87	63
Gloria	42	43	—	75	89	51
Dottie				—	71	31
Opal					—	18

Group 7	Ava	Beth	Gina	Dinah	Okie	Total
Ava	—	71	71	79	91	76
Beth		—	68	61	67	60
Gina			—	65	58	46
Dinah				—	50	37
Okie		33	42	50	—	43

Group 8	Alice	Barb	Gladys	Deb	Ona	Total
Alice	—	74	76	90	95	84
Barb		—	65	82	87	63
Gladys			—	82	93	64
Deb				—	74	33
Ona					—	14

[a]Dyads with percentage entered below the diagonal did not differ significantly ($p < .06$) in the direction of observed dominance.

TABLE A-2. Frequencies of Dyadic Dominance Behavior during Early, Middle, and End of the Observational Period

Male Groups

Group 1	Alan	Bobby	Gary	Don	Ed	Oscar	Total
Early:							
Alan	—	68	38	46	21	15	188
Bobby	46	—	45	27	30	10	158
Gary	14	13	—	32	11	3	88
Don	7	3	5	—	11	3	29
Ed	1	7	21	38	—	5	72
Oscar	2	2	1	10	0	—	15
Middle:							
Alan	—	40	26	18	52	16	152
Bobby	21	—	12	13	77	13	136
Gary	7	5	—	9	25	8	54

Group 1	Alan	Bobby	Gary	Don	Ed	Oscar	Total
Don	7	2	3	—	40	6	58
Ed	5	13	9	29	—	8	64
Oscar	7	2	1	12	23	—	45
Late:							
Alan	—	39	20	9	6	20	94
Bobby	8	—	8	8	15	13	52
Gary	2	3	—	10	5	12	32
Don	3	3	0	—	20	24	50
Ed	5	0	4	10	—	10	29
Oscar	0	1	0	7	1	—	9

Group 2	Ara	Bjorn	Gene	Doug	Ernie	Omar	Total
Early:							
Ara	—	20	2	14	17	41	94
Bjorn	19	—	8	95	16	37	175
Gene	0	2	—	1	5	1	9
Doug	4	53	4	—	15	17	93
Ernie	0	3	3	10	—	6	22
Omar	9	6	3	2	8	—	28
Middle:							
Ara	—	29	22	4	12	5	72
Bjorn	11	—	46	96	12	14	179
Gene	0	11	—	4	23	28	66
Doug	0	55	3	—	10	15	83
Ernie	0	0	10	5	—	8	23
Omar	3	1	9	0	2	—	15
Late:							
Ara	—	21	8	2	4	10	45
Bjorn	5	—	23	56	11	19	114
Gene	2	6	—	8	18	28	62
Doug	0	39	0	—	21	13	73
Ernie	0	1	6	1	—	1	9
Omar	2	1	16	3	1	—	23

Group 3	Alex	Guy	Eric	Orville	Total
Early:					
Alex	—	56	44	52	152
Guy	8	—	4	28	40
Eric	8	8	—	8	24
Orville	4	8	0	—	12
Middle:					
Alex	—	28	16	36	80
Guy	4	—	0	48	52
Eric	0	0	—	0	0
Orville	0	28	0	—	28
Late:					
Alex	—	20	5	30	55
Guy	5	—	5	65	75
Eric	0	5	—	5	10
Orville	0	40	10	—	50

Group 4	Andy	Gar	Delvin	Otto	Total
Early:					
Andy	—	57	24	74	155
Gar	—	9	15	15	37
Delvin	8	6	—	11	25
Otto	57	31	39	—	127
Middle:					
Andy	—	56	41	102	199
Gar	19	—	19	82	120
Delvin	18	17	—	83	118
Otto	36	65	69	—	170
Late:					
Andy	—	54	74	83	211
Gar	37	—	31	116	184
Delvin	20	26	—	96	142
Otto	26	48	62	—	136

Female Groups

Group 5	Amy	Betty	Gilda	Donna	Olivia	Total
Early:						
Amy	—	17	12	3	32	64
Betty	12	—	12	13	18	55
Gilda	2	11	—	12	36	61
Donna	3	3	3	—	11	20
Olivia	6	1	4	2	—	13
Middle:						
Amy	—	9	9	12	15	45
Betty	6	—	29	18	25	78
Gilda	11	15	—	21	25	72
Donna	2	2	6	—	19	29
Olivia	2	1	2	3	—	8
Late:						
Amy	—	13	6	8	7	34
Betty	3	—	24	11	23	61
Gilda	2	11	—	3	6	22
Donna	4	9	8	—	7	28
Olivia	0	4	1	0	—	5

Group 6	Ann	Becky	Gloria	Dottie	Opal	Total
Early:						
Ann	—	17	11	9	3	40
Becky	22	—	21	18	22	83
Gloria	10	18	—	8	5	41
Dottie	3	5	3	—	3	14
Opal	1	2	1	1	—	5
Middle:						
Ann	—	6	6	4	6	22
Becky	4	—	14	21	12	51
Gloria	6	10	—	3	2	21
Dottie	0	4	0	—	8	12
Opal	0	2	0	1	—	3

Group 6	Ann	Becky	Gloria	Dottie	Opal	Total
Late:						
Ann	—	24	6	25	17	72
Becky	3	—	9	13	11	36
Gloria	1	5	—	10	1	17
Dottie	3	4	4	—	18	29
Opal	2	3	0	10	—	15

Group 7	Ava	Beth	Gina	Dinah	Okie	Total
Early:						
Ava	—	11	15	17	3	46
Beth	3	—	22	22	1	48
Gina	5	9	—	9	2	25
Dinah	3	9	5	—	5	22
Okie	0	2	6	10	—	18
Middle:						
Ava	—	1	6	14	1	22
Beth	3	—	15	22	3	43
Gina	6	8	—	12	16	42
Dinah	5	10	1	—	11	27
Okie	1	0	13	23	—	37
Late:						
Ava	—	5	14	22	6	47
Beth	1	—	9	10	8	28
Gina	3	5	—	12	22	42
Dinah	6	15	12	—	25	58
Okie	0	4	10	8	—	22

Group 8	Alice	Barb	Gladys	Deb	Ona	Total
Early:						
Alice	—	38	9	51	33	131
Barb	15	—	6	34	28	83
Gladys	4	3	—	31	8	46
Deb	7	9	8	—	26	50
Ona	2	6	2	21	—	31
Middle:						
Alice	—	38	10	18	34	100
Barb	11	—	3	19	45	78
Gladys	3	6	—	15	22	46
Deb	2	6	4	—	35	47
Ona	1	7	1	3	—	12
Late:						
Alice	—	31	25	26	36	118
Barb	11	—	17	30	45	103
Gladys	7	5	—	15	37	64
Deb	2	3	1	—	32	38
Ona	2	5	2	8	—	17

Appendix B:
Middle Adolescents

TABLE B-1. Females: Frequency (N = 735) of Dyadic Dominance Interactions Between Group Members

Dominant (X)	Alice		Betty		Gretchen		Denise	
Alice	—		25	48%[a]	13	46%	37	73%**
Betty	27	52%	—		7	70%	24	62%°
Gretchen	15	54%	3	30%	—		3	50%
Denise	14	27%	15	38%	3	50%	—	
Ellen	1	33%	0	0%	4	40%	0	0%
Zoe	4	25%	0	0%	0	0%	6	33%
Theresa	3	33%	0	0%	13	50%	3	50%
Ina	0	0%	2	50%	0	0%	0	0%
Totals[c]	61	39%	45	38%	40	47%	73	59%

[a]Figures in first column under each heading indicate total frequency of recorded dominance interactions between pair in which X dominated Y; figures in second column are percentage of total dominance interactions between pair in which X dominated Y.
[b]Total number of times an individual was dominant in all pairwise interactions and percentage of total interactions in which an individual was dominant.

TABLE B-2. Males: Frequency of Dyadic Dominance Interactions Between Group Members

	Dominated (Y)					
Dominant (X)	Ben		Roger		Sam	
Group 9 (N = 879)						
Ben	—	—	74	62%[a]**	77	63%**
Roger	45	38%	—	—	39	56%
Sam	46	37%	31	44%	—	—
Ralph	34	37%	19	49%	28	39%
Tom	14	15%	6	14%	3	43%
Bill	23	23%	8	22%	6	17%
Totals[c]	162	31%	138	45%	153	50%
	Bjorn				Steve	
Group 10 (N = 705)						
Bjorn	—	—			44	60%*
Steve	29	40%			—	—
Roy	29	34%			6	22%
Pete	34	17%			15	13%
Dirk	4	9%			2	6%
Totals	96	24%			67	27%

[a]Figures in first column under each heading indicate total frequency of recorded dominance interactions between pair in which X dominated Y; figures in second column are percentage of total dominance interactions between pair in which X dominated Y.
[b]Total number of times an individual was dominant in all pairwise interactions and percentage of total interactions in which an individual was dominant.
[c]Total number of times an individual was dominated in all pairwise interactions and percentage of total interactions in which an individual was dominated.

Ellen		Zoe		Theresa		Ina		Totals[b]	
2	67%	12	75%*	6	67%	6	100%*	101	61%
4	100%°	2	100%	6	100%*	2	50%	72	62%
6	60%	5	100%*	13	50%	0	0%	45	53%
3	100%°	12	67%°	3	50%	1	100%	51	41%
—		0	0%	1	100%	29	66%*	35	52%
2	100%	—		5	83%°	8	100%**	25	35%
0	0%	1	17%	—		3	100%°	23	40%
15	34%	0	0%	0	0%	—		17	26%
32	48%	32	65%	34	60%	49	73%		

[c]Total number of times an individual was dominated in all pairwise interactions and percentage of total interactions in which an individual was dominated.
° = .15 > p < .06
* = p < .05
** = p < .01

Dominated (Y)							
Ralph		Tom		Bill		Totals[b]	
57	63%**	81	85%***	78	77%***	367	69%
20	51%	36	86%***	28	78%***	168	55%
44	61%*	4	57%	29	83%***	154	50%
—	—	10	71%°	15	71%*	106	45%
4	29%	—	—	8	57%	35	20%
6	29%	6	43%	—	—	49	24%
131	55%	137	80%	158	76%	—	—
Roy		Pete		Dirk		Totals	
56	66%**	168	83%***	41	91%***	309	76%
21	78%**	97	87%***	33	94%***	180	73%
—	—	50	86%***	20	95%***	105	55%
8	14%	—	—	32	68%**	89	21%
1	5%	15	32%	—	—	22	15%
86	45%	330	79%	126	85%	—	—

° = .15 > p < .06
* = p < .05
** = p < .01
*** = p < .001

References

Abramovitch, R. (1980). Attention structures in hierarchically organized groups. In D.R. Omark, F.F. Strayer, & D.G. Freedman (Eds.), *Dominance relations: An ethological view of human conflict and social interaction.* NY: Garland.

Adams, G.R. (1983). The study of intraindividual change during early adolescence. *The Journal of Early Adolescence, 3,* 37-46.

Adelson, J. (Ed.) (1980). *Handbook of adolescent psychology.* New York: Wiley.

Adorno, T.W., Frenkel-Brunswik, E., Levinson, D., & Stanford, R.N. (1950). *The authoritarian personality.* NY: Harper.

Aivers, C., Barnett, R., & Baruch, G. (1979). *Beyond sugar and spice: How women grow, learn, and thrive.* NY: G.P. Putman's Sons.

Alcock, J. (1975). *Animal behavior: An evolutionary approach.* Sunderland: Sinauer.

Alexander, R.D. (1974). The evolution of social behavior. *Annual Review of Ecology and Systematics, 5,* 325-383.

Alker, H.A. (1972). Is personality situationally specific or intrapsychially consistent? *Journal of Personality, 40,* 1-16.

Alston, W.P. (1975). Traits, consistency, and conceptual alternatives for personality theory. *Journal for the Theory of Social Behavior, 5,* 17-48.

Altmann, J. (1974). Observational study of behavior: Sampling methods. *Behaviour, 49,* 227-267.

Altmann, S.A. (1981). Domninance relationships: The Cheshire cat's grin. *The Behavioral and Brain Sciences, 4,* 430-431.

Anderson, H.H. (1937). Domination and integration in the social behavior of young children in an experimental play situation. *Genetic Psychology Monographs, 19,* 341-408.

Angrist, S.S. (1969). The study of sex roles. *Journal of Social Issues, 25,* 215-232.

Astrachan, A. (1984). Men: A movement of their own. *Ms,* August, 91-94.

Baenninger, R. (1981). Dominance: On distinguishing the baby from the bathwater. *The Behavioral and Brian Sciences, 4,* 431-432.

Bales, R.F. (1970). Personality and interpersonal behavior. New York: Holt, Rinehart & Winston.

Bandura, A. (1978). The self-system in reciprocal determinism. *American Psychologist, 33,* 344-358.

Banks, E.M. (1981). Dominance and behavioral primatologists: A case of typological thinking? *The Behavioral and Brain Sciences, 4,* 432-433.

Barker, R.G. & Wright, H.F. (1951). *One boy's day.* NY: Harper.

Barker, R.G. & Wright, H.F. (1955). *Midwest and its children.* New York: Harper & Row.

Bateson, P.P.G. (1968). Ethological methods of observing behavior. In L. Weiskrantz (Ed.), *Analysis of behavioral change.* NY: Harper & Row.

Bayley, N. (1965). Research in child development: A longitudinal perspective. *Merrill-Palmer Quarterly, 11,* 183-208.

Beach, F.A. (1978). Sociobiology and interspecific comparisons of behavior. In M.S. Gregory, A. Silvers, & D. Sutch (Eds.), *Sociobiology and human nature.* San Francisco: Jossey-Bass.

Bem, S.L. (1981). Gender scheme theory: A cognitive account of sex typing. *Psychological Review, 88,* 354-364.

Bem, S.L. & Lenney, E. (1976). Sex-typing and the avoidance of cross-sex behavior. *Journal of Personality and Social Psychology, 33,* 48-54.

Bem, S.L., Martyna, W., & Watson, C. (1976). Sex-typing and androgyny: Further explorations of the expressive domain. *Journal of Personality and Social Psychology, 34,* 1016-1023.

Benson, P., Dehority, J., Garman, L., Hanson, E., Hochschevender, M., Lebold, C., Rohr, R., & Sullivan, J. (1980). Intrapersonal correlates of nonspontaneous helping behavior. *Journal of Social Psychology, 110,* 87-95.

Bernstein, I.S. (1980). Dominance: A theoretical perspective for ethologists. In D.R. Omark, F.F. Strayer, & D.G. Freedman (Eds.), *Dominance relations: An ethological view of human conflict and social interaction.* NY: Garland.

Bernstein, I.S. (1981). Dominance: The baby and the bathwater. *The Behavioral and Brain Sciences, 4,* 419-429.

Berzonsky, M.D. (1983). Adolescent research: A life span developmental perspective. *Human Development, 26,* 213-221.

Block, J. (1976). Issues, problems and pitfalls in assessing sex differences: A critical review of *The psychology of sex differences. Merrill-Palmer Quarterly, 22,* 283-309.

Blos, P. (1962). *On adolescence.* New York: Free Press.

Blurton Jones, N.G. (1972). *Ethological studies of child behavior.* Cambridge: Cambridge University Press.

Blurton Jones, N.G. (1982). Editorial: Human ethology—the study of people as if they could not talk? *Ethology and Sociobiology, 2,* 51-54.

Blyth, D.A. (1986) Personal communication. Ithaca, NY.

Blyth, D.A. (1983). Moving beyond current limitations: A commentary. *The Journal of Early Adolescence, 3,* 157-162.

Boice, R. (1983). *Human ethology.* New York: Plenum.

Boice, R., Boice-Quanty, C., & Williams, R.C. (1974). Competition and possible dominance in turtles, toads, and frogs. *Journal of Comparative and Physiological Psychology, 86,* 1116-1131.

Boice, R. & Williams, R.C. (1971). Competitive feeding behavior of *Rana pipiens* and *Rana clamitans. Animal Behavior, 19,* 544-547.

Bowers, K.S. (1973). Situationism in psychology: An analysis and a critique. *Psychological Review, 80,* 307-336.

Bronfenbrenner, U. (1979). *The ecology of human development.* Cambridge, MA: Harvard University Press.

Brumberg, J.J. (in press). *Fasting girls: The emergence of anorexia nervosa.* Cambridge, MA: Harvard University Press.

Bryan, J. (1975). Children's cooperation and helping behaviors. In E.M. Hetherington (Ed.), *Review of child development research*. Volume 5. Chicago: University of Chicago Press.

Burton, R.V. (1963). Generality of honesty reconsidered. *Psychological Review, 70*, 481-499.

Buss, D.M. & Craik, K.H. (1980). The frequency concept of dispositions: Dominance and prototypically dominant acts. *Journal of Personality, 48*, 379-392.

Buss, A.H. & Plomin, R. (1984). *Temperament: Early development of personality traits.* Hillsdale, NJ: Erlbaum.

Butt, D.S. & Fiske, D.W. (1968). Comparisons of strategies in developing scales for dominance. *Psychological Bulletin, 70*, 505-519.

Cairns, R.B. (1979). *Social development: The origins and plasticity of interchanges.* San Francisco: Freeman.

California Psychological Inventory. (1964). Palo Alto: Consulting Psychologists Press.

Callan, H. (1970). *Ethology and society: Towards an anthropological view.* Oxford: Clarendon.

Campbell, D.T., & Fiske, D.W. (1959). Convergent and discriminant validation by the multitrait-multimethod matrix. *Psychological Bulletin, 56*, 81-105.

Candland, D.K., & Hoer, J.B. (1981). The logical status of dominance. *The Behavioral and Brain Sciences, 4*, 436-437.

Cantor, N. & Mischel, M. (1977). Traits as prototypes: Effects on recogntion memory. *Journal of Personality and Social Psychology, 35*, 38-48.

Chalmers, N.R. (1981). Dominance as part of a relationship. *The Behavioral and Brain Sciences, 4*, 437-438.

Chance, M.R.A. (1967). Attention structure as the basis of primate rank orders. *Man, 2*, 503-518.

Chapple, E.D. (1940). Measuring human relations: An introduction to the study of the interaction of individuals. *Genetic Psychology Monographs, 22*, 1-47.

Chase, I.D. (1981). Social interactions: The missing link in evolutionary models. *The Behavioral and Brain Sciences, 4*, 237-238.

Cheska, A. (1970). Current developments in competitive sports for girls and women. *Journal of Health, Physical Education and Recreation, 41*, 86-91.

Coleman, J.S. (1961). *The adolescent society.* Glencoe, IL: Free Press.

Coles, R. (1985a). *The moral life of children.* Boston: Atlantic Monthly Press.

Coles, R. (1985b). *The political life of children.* Boston: Atlantic Monthly Press.

Collins, B.E. & Raven, B.E. (1969). Group structure: Attraction, coalitions, communication, and power. In G. Linzey & E. Aronson (Eds.), *Handbook of social psychology, Volume 4.* Reading MA: Addison-Wesley.

Conger, J. (1971). A world they never knew: The family and social change. *Daedalus, 100*, 1105-1138.

Coombs, C. (1953). Theory and methods of social measurement. In L. Festinger & D. Katz (Eds.), *Research methods in the behavioral sciences.* NY: Holt, Rinehart & Winston.

Coopersmith, S. (1961). *The antecedents of self-esteem.* San Francisco: Freeman.

Costa, P.T. & McCrae, R.R. (1980). Still stable after all these years: Personality as a key to some issues in aging. In P.B. Baltes, O.G. Brim, Jr. (Eds.), *Life-span development and behavior,* Vol. 3, NY: Academic Press.

Cronbach, L.J. (1975). Beyond the two disciplines of scientific psychology. *American Psychologist, 30,* 116-127.

Cronin, C.L. (1975). The place of girls in the social structure of children's groups. Unpublished manuscript, University of Chicago.

Csikszentmihalyi, M. & Larson, R. (1984). *Being adolescent.* New York: Basic Books.

Darwin, C. (1872). *The expression of emotions in man and animals.* London: D. Appleton.

David, D.S. & Brannon, R. (Eds.) (1976). *The forty-nine percent majority: The male sex role.* Boston: Addison-Wesley.

Dawkins, R. (1976). *The selfish gene.* NY: Oxford University Press.

Dlugokinski, E.L. & Firestone, I.J. (1973). Congruence among four methods of measuring other centeredness. *Child Development, 44,* 304-308.

Dolhinow, P. (1972). *Primate Patterns.* NY: Holt, Rinehart & Winston.

Douvan, E. (1960). Sex differences in adolescent character processes. *Merrill-Palmer Quarterly, 6,* 203-211.

Douvan, E., & Adelson, J. (1966). *The adolescent experience.* NY: Wiley.

Dumont, L. (1970). *Homo hierarchicus: An essay on the caste system.* Chicago: University of Chicago Press.

Eibl-Eibesfeldt, I. (1975). *Ethology: The biology of behavior,* revised edition. NY: Holt, Rinehart & Winston.

Eibl-Eibesfeldt, I. (1979). Human ethology: Concepts and implications for the sciences of man. *The Behavioral and Brain Sciences, 2,* 1-26.

Eibl-Eibesfeldt, I. (1985). On the aims of our organization. *Human Ethology Newsletter, 4*(issue 7), 1-3.

Eisenberg-Berg, N., & Lennon, R. (1980). Altruism and the assessment of empathy in the preschool years. *Child Development, 51,* 552-557.

Elder, G. Jr. (1980). Adolescence in historical perspective. In J. Adelson (Ed.), *Handbook of adolescent psychology.* New York: Wiley.

Elkins, H. (1978). Time for a change: Women's athletics and the women's movement. *Frontiers, 3,* 22-25.

Ellyson, S.L. & Dovidio, J.F. (1985). *Power, dominance, and nonverbal behavior.* NY: Springer-Verlag.

Endler, N.S. (1975). The case for person-situation interactions. *Canadian Psychological Review, 16,* 12-21.

Endler, N.S. & Magnusson, D. (1976). Toward an interactional psychology of personality. *Psychological Bulletin, 83,* 956-974.

Epstein, S. (1979). The stability of behavior I: On predicting most of the people much of the time. *Journal of Personality and Social Psychology, 37,* 1097-1126.

Epstein, S. (1980). The stability of behavior II: Implications for psychological research. *American Psychologist, 35,* 790-806.

Erikson, E.H. (1959). Identity and the life cycle. *Psychological Issues, 1,* 1-171.

Esser, A.H. (1973). Cottage Fourteen: Dominance and territoriality in a group of institutionalized boys. *Small Group Behavior, 4,* 131-146.

Farrell, W. (1974). *The liberated man.* NY: Random House.

Felshin, J. (1973). The social anomaly of women in sports. *The Physical Educator, 30,* 122-123.

Fine, G.A. & Glassner, B. (1979). Participant observation with children: Promise and problems. *Urban Life, 8,* 153-174.

Flannelly, K.J. & Blanchard, R.J. (1981). Dominance: Cause or description of social relationships? *The Behavioral and Brain Sciences, 4,* 438-440.

Freedman, D.G. (1974). *Human infancy: An evolutionary perspective.* NY: Halstead.

Freedman, D.G. (1979). *Human sociobiology: A holistic approach.* NY: Free Press.

Friedenberg, E. Z. (1959). *The vanishing adolescent.* Boston: Beacon Press.

Friedrich, L.K., & Stein, A.H. (1973). Aggressive and prosocial television programs and the natural behavior of preschool children. *Monographs of the Society for Research in Child Development, 38,* (4, Serial no. 151).

Gallagher, J.R. & Brouha, L. (1943). A simple method of testing the physical fitness of boys. *Research Quarterly, 14,* 23-31.

Gage, F.H. (1981). Dominance: Measure first and then define. *The Behavioral and Brain Sciences, 4,* 440-441.

Gartlan, J.S. (1964). Dominance in East African monkeys. *Proceedings of the East African Academy, 2,* 75-79.

Gauthreaux, S.A., Jr. (1981). Behavioral dominance from an ecological perspective. *The Behavioral and Brain Sciences, 4,* 441.

Gellert, E. (1961). Stability and fluctuation in the power relationships of young children. *Journal of Abnormal and Social Psychology, 62,* 8-15.

Gibb, C.A. (1969). Leadership. In G. Linzey & E. Aronson (Eds.), *Handbook of social psychology, Volume 4.* Cambridge, MA: Addison-Wesley.

Gifford, R. (1982). Affiliativeness: A trait measure in relation to single-act and multiple-act behavioral criteria. *Journal of Research in Personality, 16,* 128-134.

Gilligan, C. (1982). *In a different voice: Psychological theory and women's development.* Cambridge, MA: Harvard University Press.

Glidewell, J.C., Kantor, M.B., Smith, L.M., & Stringer, L.A. (1966). Socialization and social structures in the classroom. In L.W. Hoffman & M.L. Hoffman (Eds.), *Review of child development research.* NY: Russell Sage.

Golding, W. (1954). *Lord of the flies.* NY: Capricorn Books.

Goodall, J. (1968). The behavior of free-living chimpanzees in the Gombe Stream Reserve. *Animal Behaviour Monographs, 1,* 161-311.

Gordon, M.H., Loveland, E.H., & Cureton, E.E. (1952). An extended table of chi-square for two degrees of freedom, for use in combining probabilities from independent samples. *Psychometrika, 17,* 311-316.

Gottman, J.M. & Ringland, J.T. (1981). The analysis of dominance and bidirectionality in social development. *Child Development, 52,* 393-412.

Grinder, R.E. (1967). *A history of genetic psychology.* New York: Wiley.

Grinder, R.E. (1982). Isolationism in adolescent research. *Human Development, 25,* 223-232.

Guthrie, R. (1970). Evolution of human threat display organs. In T. Dobzhansky, M.K. Hecht & W.C. Steere (Eds.), *Evolutionary biology.* NY: Appleton-Century-Crofts.

Hall, E.T. (1966) *The hidden dimension.* NY: Doubleday.

Hall, G.S. (1904). *Adolescence: Its psychology and its relations to physiology, anthropology, sociology, sex, crime, religion, and education.* New York: Appleton.

Hamilton, S.F. (In preparation). Becoming a worker: The transition from school to work in the United States and West Germany.

Hartshorne, H., May, M.A., & Maller, J.B. (1929). *Studies in service and self-control.* NY: MacMillan.

Hartup, W.W. (1983). Peer relations. In P.H. Mussen (Ed.-in-Chief) & E.M. Hetherington (volume editor), *Handbook of child psychology,* 4th edition,

Volume IV: Socialization, personality, and social development. New York: Wiley.

Hartup, W.W. & Keller, E. (1960). Nurturance in preschool children and its relation to dependency. *Child Development, 31,* 681-689.

Harvard Computation Laboratory Staff. (1955). *Tables of the cumulative binomial probability distribution.* Cambridge, MA: Harvard University Press.

Hicks, B. (1979). Lesbian athletes. *Christopher Street* (October), 42-50.

Hill, J.P. (1982).Guest editorial. *Child Development, 53,* 1409-1412.

Hill, J.P. (1983). Early adolescence: A research agenda. *The Journal of Early Adolescence, 3,* 1-21.

Hinde, R.A. (1966). *Animal behaviour: A synthesis of ethology and comparative psychology.* NY: McGraw-Hill.

Hinde, R.A. & Datta, S. (1981). Dominance: An intervening variable. *The Behavioral and Brain Sciences, 4,* 442.

Hoffman, M. (1979). Development of moral thought, feeling and behavior. *American Psychologist, 84,* 712-720.

Holden, C. (1980). Twins united. *Science 80,* (November), 55-59.

Hollingshead, A.B. (1949). *Elmtown's youth.* New York: Wiley.

Hollingshead, A.B. (1975) *Elmtown's youth and Elmtown revisited.* NY: Wiley.

Holstein, C. (1976). Development of moral judgment: A longitudinal study of males and females. *Child Development, 47,* 51-61.

Hrdy, S.B. (1981). *The woman that never evolved.* Cambridge, MA: Harvard University Press.

Hutt, C. (1972). *Males and females.* Baltimore: Penguin.

Itani, J. (1961). The society of Japanese monkeys. *Japan Quarterly, 8,* 1-10.

Jaccard, J.J. (1974). Predicting social behavior from personality traits. *Journal of Research in Personality, 7,* 358-367.

Jay, S.M. & Elliott, C. (1984). Behavioral observation scales for measuring children's distress: The effects of increased methodological rigor. *Journal of Consulting and Clinical Psychology, 52,* 1106-1107.

Johnson, W.R., & Coffer, C.V. (1974). Personality dynamics: Psychosocial implications. In W.R. Johnson & E.R. Buskirk (Eds.), *Science and medicine of exercise and sport.* NY: Harper & Row.

Jones, E.E., & Nisbet, R.E. (1972). The actor and the observer: Divergent perceptions of the causes of behavior. In E.E. Jones et al. (Eds.), *Attribution: Perceiving the causes of behavior.* Morristown, NJ: General Learning Press.

Jones, H.E. (1958). Problems of method in longitudinal research. *Vita Humana, 1,* 93-99.

Jones, L.V. & Fiske, D.W. (1953). Models for testing the significance of combined results. *Psychological Bulletin, 50,* 375-382.

Jorgensen, S.R. (1983). Beyond adolescent pregnancy: Research frontiers for early adolescent sexuality. *The Journal of Early Adolescence, 3,* 141-155.

Kandel, D. & Lesser, G. (1972). *Youth in two worlds.* San Francisco: Jossey-Bass.

Kaplan, A. (1971). The effects of sex and dominance on three dimensions of children's interactions. Unpublished manuscript, University of Chicago.

Kaplan, J.R. (1981). A reexamination of dominance rank and hierarchy in primates. *The Behavioral and Brain Sciences, 4,* 442-443.

Katchadourian, H. (1977). *The biology of adolescence.* San Francisco: W.H. Freeman.

Katz, P. (1979). The development of female identity. *Sex Roles, 5,* 155-178.

Kelley, H.H. (1952). Two functions of reference groups. In T.M. Newcomb & E.L.

Hartley (Eds.), *Readings in social psychology,* revised edition. NY: Holt, Rinehart & Winston.

Kett, J. (1977). *Rites of passage: Adolescence in America, 1790 to the present.* New York: Basic Books.

Kiell, N. (1964). *The universal experience of adolescence.* New York: International Universities Press.

Klissouras, V. (1984). Factors affecting physical performance with reference to heredity. In J. Borms and associates (Eds.), *Human growth and development.* NY: Plenum.

Koslin, B.L., Harrlow, R.N., Karlins, M. & Pargament, R. (1968). Predicting group status from members' cognition. *Sociometry, 31,* 64-75.

Kreuz, L.E., Rose, R.M., & Jennings, J.R. (1972). Suppression of plasma testosterone levels and psychological stress. *Archives of General Psychiatry, 26,* 479-482.

Lacoste-Utamsing, C. de & Holloway, R.L. (1982) Sexual dimorphism in the human corpus callosum. *Science, 216,* 1431-1432.

Lamiell, J.T. (1981). Toward an idiothetic psychology of personality. *American Psychologist, 36,* 276-284.

Lancaster, J.B. (1984). Introduction. In M.F. Small (Ed.), *Female primates: Studies by women primatologists.* NY: Alan R. Liss.

Latane, B., & Darley, J. (1970). *The unresponsive bystander: Why doesn't he help?* NY: Appleton-Century-Crofts.

Leeds, A. (1984). Sociobiology, anti-sociobiology, epistemology, and human nature. In R.S. Cohen & M.W. Wartofsky (Eds.), *Methodology, metaphysics and the history of science.* Dordrecht, Holland: D. Reidel.

Lerner, R.M. (1981). Adolescent development: Scientific study in the 1980s. *Youth and Society, 12,* 251-275.

Lewontin, R.C., Rose, S., & Kamin, L.J. (1984). *Not in our genes: Biology, ideology and human nature.* NY: Pantheon.

Levi-Strauss, C. (1951). *Tristes tropiques.* Translated by J. Russell. NY: Criterion Books.

Lippitt, R. & Gold, M. (1959). Classroom social structure as a mental health problem. *Journal of Social Issues, 15,* 40-49.

Lippitt, R., Polansky, N. & Rosen, S. (1952). The dynamics of power: A field study of social influence in groups of children. *Human Relations, 5,* 37-64.

Livson, N. & Peskin, H. (1980). Perspectives on adolescence from longitudinal research. In J. Adelson (Ed.), *Handbook of adolescent psychology.* New York: Wiley.

Loizos, C. (1969). An ethological study of chimpanzee play. In C.R. Carpenter (Ed.), *Proceedings of the 2nd International Congress of Primatology, Volume 1, Behavior.* NY: S. Karger.

Lorenz, K.Z. (1935). Oer kumpon in der umwelt des vogels. *Journal of Ornithology, 83,* 137-413.

Lorenz, K.Z. (1966). *On aggression.* NY: Harcourt, Brace, & World.

Lott, D.F. (1981). Circumstances in which exact dominance rank may be important. *The Behavioral and Brain Sciences, 4,* 443-444.

Loy, J.W., McPherson, D., & Kenyon, G. (1978). *Sport and social systems.* Reading, MA: Addison-Wesley.

Maccoby, E.E. & Jacklin, C.N. (1974). *The psychology of sex differences.* Stanford: Stanford University Press.

MacDonald, K.B. (1986). Biological and psychosocial interactions in early adolescence: A sociobiological perspective. In R.M. Lerner & T.T. Foch (Eds.), *Biological and psychosocial interactions in early adolescence: A lifespan perspective.* Hillsdale, NJ: Erlbaum.

MacDonald, K.B. (Ed.) (In preparation). *Sociobiological perspectives on human development.*

Magnusson, D. & Endler, N.S. (Eds.) (1977). *Personality at the crossroads: Current issues in interactional psychology.* Hillsdale, NJ: Erlbaum.

Masters, R.D. (1984). Ostracism, voice, and exit: The biology of social participation. *Social Science Information, 23,* 877-893.

Matza, D. (1964). Position and behavior patterns of youth. In J. Faris (Ed.), *Handbook of modern sociology.* Chicago: Rand McNally.

Maxim, P.E. (1981). Dominance: A useful dimension of social communication. *The Behavioral and Brain Sciences, 4,* 444-445.

Mazur, A., Mazur, J., & Keating, C. (1984). Military rank attainment of a West Point class: Effects of cadets' physical features. *American Journal of Sociology, 90,* 125-150.

McCall, R. (1977). Challenges to a science of developmental psychology. *Child Development, 48,* 333-344.

McGrew, W.C. (1972). *An ethological study of children's behavior.* NY: Academic Press.

McGuinness, D. (1984). The emotions: Focus on intermale aggression and dominance systems. In *Absolute values and the new cultural revolution.* Twelfth International Conference on the Unity of the Sciences, Chicago, IL. NY: I.C.U.S. Books.

McGuinness, D. (Ed.) (in press). *Dominance and inter-male aggression.* NY: Paragon.

McGuire, M.T. (1974). The St. Kitts vervet. In H. Kuhn (Ed.), *Contributions to primatology, Volume 2.* Basel, Switzerland: S. Karger.

Mead, G.H. (1934). *Mind, self and society.* Chicago: University of Chicago Press.

Mead, M. (1928). *Coming of age in Samoa.* New York: Morrow.

Medin, D.L. (1974). The comparative study of memory. *Journal of Human Evolution, 3,* 455-463.

Meek, L.H. (1940). *The personal-social development of boys and girls with implications for secondary education.* NY: Progressive Education Association.

Mischel, W. (1968). *Personality and assessment.* NY: Wiley.

Mischel, W. (1977). On the future of personality measurement. *American Psychologist, 32,* 246-254.

Mitchell, G. & Brandt, E.M. (1972). Paternal behavior in primates. In F.E. Poirier (Ed.), *Primate socialization.* NY: Random House.

Mussen, P., & Eisenberg-Berg, N. (1977). *Roots of caring, sharing and helping.* San Francisco: W.H. Freeman.

Mussen, P. & Jones, M.C. (1957). Self-conceptions, motivations, and interpersonal attitudes of late-and early-maturing boys. *Child Development, 28,* 243-256.

Offer, D. (1969). *The psychological world of the teenager.* New York: Basic Books.

Olweus, D. (1977). Aggression and peer acceptance in adolescent boys: Two short-term longitudinal studies of ratings. *Child Development, 48,* 1301-1313.

Omark, D.R. (1980). Human ethology: A holistic perspective. In D.R. Omark, F.F. Strayer, & D.G. Freedman (Eds.), *Dominance relations: An ethological view of human conflict and social interaction.* NY: Garland.

Omark, D.R. & Edelman, M.S. (1976). The development of attention structure in young children. In M.R.A. Chance & R.R. Larson (Eds.), *The structure of social attention*. NY: Wiley.

Omark, D.R., Strayer, F.F., & Freedman, D.G. (Eds.) (1980). *Dominance relations: An ethological view of human conflict and social interaction*. New York: Garland.

Orne, M.T. (1973). Communication by the total experimental situation: Why it is important, how it is evaluated, and its significance for ecological validity of findings. In P. Pliner, L. Krames, & T. Alloway (Eds.), *Communication and affect*. NY: Academic Press.

Paikoff, R.L. & Savin-Williams, R.C. (1983). An exploratory study of dominance interactions among adolescent females at a summer camp. *Journal of Youth and Adolescence, 12,* 419-433.

Parsons, T. & Bales, R.F. (1955). *Family, socialization, and interaction process*. Glencoe, IL: The Free Press.

Pattee, H.H. (1973). *Hierarchy theory: The challenge of complex systems*. NY: George Braziller.

Peskin, H. (1973). Influence of the developmental schedule of puberty on learning and ego functioning. *Journal of Youth and Adolescence, 2,* 273-290.

Petersen, A.C., Tobin-Richards, M. & Boxer, A. (1983). Puberty: Its measurement and its meaning. *The Journal of Early Adolescence, 3,* 47-62.

Pitcairn, T.K., & Strayer, F.F. (1984). Social attention and group structure: Variations on Schubert's "Winterreise." *Journal of Social and Biological Structure, 7,* 369-376.

Pleck, J.H. (1981). *The myth of masculinity*. Cambridge, MA: MIT Press.

Poirier, F.E. (1974). Colobine aggression: A review. In R.L. Holloway (Ed.), *Primate aggression, territoriality, and xenophobia*. NY: Academic Press.

Polansky, N.W., Freeman, M., Horowitz, L., Irwin, N., Papania, D., Rapaport, D. & Whaley, F. (1949). Problems of interpersonal relations in research on groups. *Human Relations, 2,* 281-291.

Polsky, H.W. (1962). *Cottage six: The social system of delinquent boys in residential treatment*. NY: Wiley.

Postman, N. (1986). A singer of their tales. *New York Times Book Review,* January 19, pp. 1 & 28.

Radke-Yarrow, M., Zahn-Waxler, C., & Chapman, M. (1983). Children's prosocial dispositions and behavior. In P.M. Mussen (Ed.-in-Chief) and E.M. Hetherington, (Ed.), *Carmichael's manual of child psychology,* 4th edition, *Volume 4.* NY: Wiley.

Ramirez, J.M. & Mendoza, D.L. (1984). Gender differences in social interactions of children: A naturalistic approach. *Bulletin of the Psychonomic Society, 22,* 553-556.

Redican, W.K. & Taub, D.M. (1981). Male parental care in monkeys and apes. In M.E. Lamb (Ed.), *The role of the father in child development,* 2nd edition. NY: Wiley.

Richards, S.M. (1974). The concept of dominance and methods of assessment. *Animal Behaviour, 22,* 914-930.

Riesen, A.H. (1974). Comparative perspectives in behavior study. *Journal of Human Evolution, 3,* 433-434.

Roberts, J.M., & Sutton-Smith, B. (1962). Child training and game involvement. *Ethnology, 1,* 166-185.

Robinson, J. & Shaver, P. (1973). *Measures of social psychological attitudes.* Ann Arbor MI: Institute for Social Research.

Romer, N. (1981). *Sex role cycle.* NY: McGraw-Hill.

Rosenblum, L.A., Coe, C.L. & Bromley, L.J. (1975). Peer relations in monkeys: The influence of social structure, gender, and familiarity. In M. Lewis and L.A. Rosenblum (Eds.), *The origins of behavior: Peer relations and friendships.* NY: Wiley.

Rowell, T.E. (1966). Hierarchy in the organization of a captive baboon group. *Animal Behaviour, 14,* 430-443.

Rowell, T.E. (1974). The concept of social dominance. *Behavioral Biology, 11,* 131-154.

Rushton, J.P. (1980). *Altruism, socialization and society.* Englewood Cliffs, NJ: Prentice-Hall.

Rushton, J.P., Brainerd, C.J. & Pressley, M. (1983) Behavioral development and construct validity: The principle of aggregation. *Psychological Bulletin, 94,* 18-38.

Rushton, J.P., Chrisjohn, R.D.,& Fekken, G.C. (1981). The altruistic personality and the self-report altruism scale. *Personality and Individual Differences, 2,* 293-302.

Rushton, J.P., Fulker, D.W., Neale, M.C., Blizard, R.A. & Eysenck, H.J. (1984). Altruism and genetics. *Acta Geneticae Medicae et Gemellologiae, 33,* 265-271.

Sade, D.S. (1967). Determinants of dominance in a group of free-ranging rhesus monkeys. In S.A. Altmann (Ed.), *Social communication among primates.* Chicago: University of Chicago Press.

Sade, D.S. (1981). Patterning of aggression. *The Behavioral and Brain Sciences, 4,* 446-447.

Sassen, G. (1980). Success anxiety in women: A constructivist interpretation of its sources and its significance. *Harvard Educational Review, 50,* 13-25.

Savin-Williams, R.C. (1976). An ethological study of dominance formation and maintenance in a group of human adolescents. *Child Development, 47,* 972-979.

Savin-Williams, R.C. (1977). Dominance in a human adolescent group. *Animal Behaviour, 25,* 400-406.

Savin-Williams, R.C. (1979). Dominance hierarchies in groups of early adolescents. *Child Development, 50,* 923-935.

Savin-Williams, R.C. (1980a). Dominance and submission among adolescent boys. In D.R. Omark, F.F. Strayer, & D.G. Freedman (Eds.), *Dominance relations: An ethological view of human conflict and social interaction.* NY: Garland.

Savin-Williams, R.C. (1980b). Social interactions of adolescent females in natural groups. In H. Foot, T. Chapman & J. Smith (Eds.) *Friendship and social relations in children.* London: Wiley.

Savin-Williams, R.C. (1980c). Dominance hierarchies in groups of middle to late adolescent males. *Journal of Youth and Adolescence, 9,* 75-87.

Savin-Williams, R.C. (1982). A field study of adolescent social interactions: Developmental and contextual influences. *Journal of Social Psychology, 117,* 203-209.

Savin-Williams, R.C. (in press). Dominance systems among primate adolescents. In D. McGuinness (Ed.), *Dominance and inter-male aggression.* NY: Paragon.

Savin-Williams, R.C., Bolger, N. & Spinola, S.M. (1986). Social interactions of adolescent girls during sports activity: Age and sex role influences. *The Journal of Early Adolescence, 6,* 67-75.

Savin-Williams, R.C. & Demo, D.H. (1983). Conceiving or misconceiving the self: Issues in adolescent self-esteem. *The Journal of Early Adolescence, 3,* 121-140.

Savin-Williams, R.C. & Freedman, D.G. (1977). Bio-social approach to human development. In S. Chevalier-Skolnikoff & F.E. Poirer (Eds.), *Primate bio-social development: Biological, social and ecological determinants.* NY: Garland.

Savin-Williams, R.C. & Jaquish, G.A. (1981). The assessment of adolescent self-esteem: A comparison of methods. *Journal of Personality, 49,* 324-336.

Savin-Williams, R.C., Small, S.A. & Zeldin, R.S. (1981). Dominance and altruism among adolescent males: A comparison of ethological and psychological methods. *Ethology and Sociobiology, 2,* 167-176.

Scheinfeld, D.R. (1973). *Dominance, exchange and achievement in a lower income Black neighborhood.* Unpublished doctoral dissertation, University of Chicago.

Schneirla, T.C. (1951). The "levels" concept in the study of social organization in animals. In J.H. Rohrer & M. Sherif (Eds.), *Social psychology at the crossroads.* NY: Harper.

Schoggen, P. (1978). Ecological psychology and mental retardation. In G.P. Sackett (Ed.), *Observing behavior, Volume 1: Theory and applications in mental retardation.* Baltimore: University Park Press.

Schoggen, P.S. (1986). Personal communication. Ithaca, NY.

Schwartz, S. (1986). Words, deeds, and the perception of consequences and responsibility in action situations. *Journal of Personality and Social Psychology, 12,* 232-242.

Scott, J.P. (1953). Implications of infra-human social behavior for problems of human relations. In M. Sherif & M.O. Wilson (Eds.), *Groups relations at the crossroads.* NY: Harper.

Seyfarth, R.M. (1981). Do monkeys rank each other? *The Behavioral and Brain Sciences, 4,* 447-448.

Shaw, C.R. (1930). *The jack-roller.* Chicago: The University of Chicago Press.

Sherif, M., Harvey, O.J., White, B.J., Hood, W.R., & Sherif, C.W. (1961). *Intergroup conflict and cooperation: The robbers cave experiment.* Norman, OK: Institute of Group Relations.

Sherif, C.W., Kelly, M., Rodgers, H.L., Sarup, G., & Tittler, B. (1973). Personal involvement, social judgment and action. *Journal of Personality and Social Psychology, 27,* 311-328.

Sherif, M. & Sherif, C.W. (1953). *Groups in harmony and tension.* New York: Harper.

Sherif, M. & Sherif, C.W. (1964). *Reference groups.* Chicago: Regnery.

Shweder, R.A. (1975). How relevant is an individual differences theory of personality? *Journal of Personality, 43,* 455-484.

Siegel, S. (1956). *Nonparametric statistics for the behavioral sciences.* NY: McGraw-Hill.

Small, M.F. (1984). *Female primates: Studies by women primatologists. Volume 4, Monographs in primatology.* NY: Alan R. Liss.

Small, S.A., Savin-Williams, R.C. & Zeldon, R.S. (1983). In search of personality traits: A multimethod analysis of naturally occurring prosocial and dominance behavior. *Journal of Personality, 51,* 1-16.

Smuts, B. (1981). Dominance: An alternative view. *The Behavioral and Brain Sciences, 4,* 448-449.

Snyder, E.E. & Kivlin, J.E. (1977). Perceptions of the sex role among female athletes and nonathletes. *Adolescence, 12,* 23-29.

Snyder, E.E., & Spreitzer, E. (1973). Family influence and involvement in sport. *Research Quarterly, 44,* 249-255.

Sommer, R. (1977). Toward a psychology of natural behavior. *APA Monitor, 8,* 1 & 7.

Southwick, C.M. (1972). Aggression among non-human primates. *Module, 23,* 1-23.

Staub, E. (1978). *Positive social behavior and morality, Volume I: Social and personal influences.* NY: Academic Press.

Staub, E. (1979). *Positive social behavior and morality, Volume 2: Socialization and development.* NY: Academic Press.

Steinberg, L.D. (1981). Transformations in family relations at puberty. *Developmental Psychology, 17,* 833-840.

Strayer, F.F. (1980). Current problems in the study of human dominance. In D.R. Omark, F.F. Strayer, & D.G. Freedman (Eds.), *Dominance relations: An ethological view of human conflict and social interaction.* NY: Garland.

Strayer, F.F., Wareing, S., & Rushton, J.P. (1979). Social constraints on naturally occurring preschool altruism. *Ethology and Sociobiology, 1,* 3-11.

Suttles, C.D. (1968). *The social order of the slum.* Chicago: University of Chicago Press.

Swartz, K.B., & Rosenblum, L.A. (1981). The social context of parental behavior. In D.J. Gubernick & P.H. Klopfer (Eds.), *Parental care in mammals.* NY: Plenum.

Syme, G.J. (1974). Competitive orders as measures of social dominance. *Animal Behaviour, 22,* 931-940.

Symons, D. (1979). *The evolution of human sexuality.* NY: Oxford University Press.

Tanner, J.M. (1962). *Growth at adolescence, 2nd edition.* Oxford: Blackwell Scientific Publications.

Taylor, J. & Reitz, W. (1968). The three faces of self-esteem. *Research Bulletin* No. 80, Department of Psychology, University of Western Ontario.

Thompson, C. (1985). You fag! Working with adolescents around homophobia. Presentation at Planned Parenthood of Tompkins County Workshop, Ithaca, NY.

Thompson, P.R. (1975). A cross-species analysis of carnivore, primate, and hominid behaviour. *Journal of Human Evolution, 4,* 113-124.

Thornburg, H.D. & Thornburg, E.E. (Eds.) (1983). Early adolescence: Research agenda for the 1980s. *The Journal of Early Adolescence, 3,* Numbers 1 & 2.

Thrasher, F. (1927). *The gang.* Chicago: University of Chicago Press.

Tiger, L. (1969). *Men in groups.* NY: Random House.

Tiger, L. (1970). Dominance in human socieities. *Annual Review of Ecology and Systematics, 1,* 287-306.

Tinbergen, N. (1953). *Social behaviour in animals.* London: Methuen.

Tinbergen, N. (1963). On aims and methods of ethology. *Zeitschrift fur Tier-psychologie, 20,* 410-433.

Tinbergen, N. (1968). On war and peace in animals and man. *Science, 160,* 1411-1418.

Torrance, E.P. (1966). *Thinking creatively with words.* Princeton, NJ: Personnel.

Trivers, R.L. (1971). The evolution of reciprocal altruisms. *Quarterly Review of Biology, 46,* 35-57.

Udry, J.R., Billy, J.O.G., Morris, N.M., Groff, T.R., & Raj, M.H. (1985). Serum androgenic hormones motivate sexual behavior in adolescent boys. *Fertility and Sterility, 43,* 90-94.

Urberg, K., & Labouvie-Vief, G. (1976). Conceptualizations of sex roles: A life-span developmental study. *Developmental Psychology, 12,* 15-23.

Vaughn, B.E. & Waters, E. (1980). Social organization among preschool peers: Dominance, attention, and sociometric correlates. In D.R. Omark, F.F. Strayer, & D.G. Freedman (Eds.), *Dominance relations: An ethological view of human conflict and social interaction.* NY: Garland.

Washburn, S.L. & Hamburg, D.A. (1968). The implications of primate research. In I. DeVore (Ed.), *Primate behavior.* NY: Holt, Rinehart, & Winston.

Webb, E., Campbell, D., Schwartz, R. & Sechrest, L. (1966). *Unobtrusive measures: Nonreactional research in the social sciences.* Chicago: Rand McNally.

Wechsler, D. (1965). *Manual of the Wechsler Intelligence Scale for Children ages 5-15.* NY: Psychological Corp.

Weisfeld, C.C., Weisfeld, G.E. & Callaghan, J.W. (1982). Female inhibition in mixed-sex competition among young adolescents. *Ethology and Sociobiology, 3,* 29-42.

Weisfeld, G.E. (1979). An ethological view of human adolescence. *The Journal of Nervous and Mental Disease, 167,* 38-55.

Weisfeld, G.E. & Berger, J.M. (1983). Some features of human adolescence viewed in evolutionary perspective. *Human Development, 26,* 121-133.

Weisfeld, G.E., Bloch, S.A. & Ivers, J.W. (1984). Possible determinants of social dominance among adolescent girls. *Journal of Genetic Psychology, 144,* 115-129.

Weisfeld, G.E., & Linkey, H.E. (1985). Dominance displays as indicators of a social success motive. In S.L. Ellyson & J.F. Dovidio (Eds.), *Power, dominance, and nonverbal behavior.* NY: Springer-Verlag.

Weisfeld, G.E., Muczenski, D.M. Weisfeld, C.C., & Omark, D.R. (In preparation). Stability of boys' social success among peers over an eleven-year period.

Weisfeld, G.E., Omark, D.R., & Cronin, C.L. (1980). A longitudinal and cross-sectional study of dominance in boys. In D.R. Omark, F.F. Strayer, & D.G. Freedman (Eds.), *Dominance relations: An ethological view of human conflict and social interaction.* NY: Garland.

Weisfeld, G.E. & Weisfeld, C.C. (1984). An observational study of social evaluation: An application of the dominance hierarchy model. *Journal of Genetic Psychology, 145,* 89-100.

Wells, L.E. & Marwell, G. (1976). *Self-esteem: Its conceptualization and measurement.* Beverly Hills, CA: Sage.

Whiting, B. & Edwards, C.P. (1973). A cross-cultural analysis of sex differences in the behavior of children aged three through eleven. *Journal of Social Psychology, 91,* 171-188.

Whyte, L.L., Wilson, A.F., & Wilson, D. (1969). *Hierarchical structures.* NY: American Elsevier.

Wickler, W. (1967). Socio-sexual signals and their intra-specific imitation among primates. In D. Morris (Ed.), *Primates ecology.* Chicago: Aldine.

Wilson, E.O. (1975). *Sociobiology: The new synthesis.* Cambridge, MA: Harvard University Press.

Wilson, M. & Daly, M. (1985). Competitiveness, risk taking, and violence: The young male syndrome. *Ethology and Sociobiology, 6,* 59-73.

Wright, H.F. (1960). Observational child study. In P. Mussen (Ed.), *Handbook of research methods in child development.* NY: Wiley.

Yarrow, M.R., Waxler, C.Z., & associates. (1976). Dimensions and correlates of prosocial behavior in young children. *Child Development, 47,* 118-125.

Yoshiba, K. (1968). Local and intertroop variability in ecology and social behavior of common Indian langurs. In P.C. Jay (Ed.), *Primates.* NY: Holt, Rinehart, & Winston.

Zahn-Waxler, C., Radke-Yarrow, M., & King, R. (1979). Child-rearing and children's initiations towards victims of distress. *Child Development, 50,* 319-330.

Zarit, S. (1970). Some aspects of the child's social world. Unpublished manuscript, The University of Chicago.

Zeldin, R.S., Savin-Williams, R.C., & Small, S.A. (1984). Dimensions of prosocial behavior in adolescent males. *The Journal of Social Psychology, 123,* 159-168.

Zeldin, R.S., Small, S.A., & Savin-Williams, R.C. (1982). Prosocial interactions in two mixed-sex adolescent groups. *Child Development, 53,* 1492-1498.

Zuckerman, S. (1932). *The social life of monkeys and apes.* London: Kegan Paul.

Author Index

Abramovitch, R., 149, 213
Adams, G.R., 3, 4, 5, 213
Adelson, J., viii, 2, 123, 213, 216
Adorno, T.W., 22, 213
Aivers, C., 144, 213
Alcock, J., 30, 213
Alexander, R.D., 33, 200, 202, 213
Alker, H.A., 173, 213
Alston, W.P., 177, 213
Altmann, J., 41, 213
Altmann, S.A., 29, 213
Anderson, H.H., 23, 213
Angrist, S.S., 128, 129, 213
Astrachan, A., 207, 213

Baenninger, R., 31, 213
Bales, R.F., 23, 150, 213, 221
Bandura, A., 5, 213
Banks, E.M., 34, 213
Barker, R.G., 9, 26, 211, 214
Barnett, R., 144, 213
Baruch, G., 144, 213
Bateson, P.P.G., 25, 214
Bayley, N., 10, 11, 214
Beach, F.A., 14, 26, 214
Bem, S.L., 146, 147, 214
Benson, P., 196, 214
Berger, J.M., 15, 157, 225
Bernstein, I.S., 27, 28, 29, 30, 31, 32,
    33, 34, 40, 41, 113, 119, 131, 173,
    185, 186, 194, 199, 214
Berzonsky, M.D., 1, 3, 5, 6, 173, 214
Billy, J.O.G., 13, 205, 225
Blanchard, R.J., 28, 217
Blizard, R.A., 181, 222

Bloch, S.A., 123, 151, 225
Block, J., 158, 214
Blos, P., viii
Blurton-Jones, N.G., 24, 26, 46, 214
Blyth, D.A., 2, 3, 4, 5, 7, 13, 173, 214
Boice, R., ix, 14, 17, 24, 214
Boice-Quanty, C., 17, 214
Bolger, N., 144, 223
Bowers, K.S., 173, 214
Boxer, A., 4, 5, 221
Brainerd, C.J., 181, 222
Brandt, E.M., 25, 220
Brannon, R., 208, 216
Bromley, L.J., 25, 222
Bronfenbrenner, U., 5, 195, 196, 214
Brouha, L., 47, 217
Brumberg, J.J., 2, 214
Bryan, J., 158, 215
Burton, R.V., 174, 215
Buss, A.H., 173, 215
Buss, D.M., 173, 177, 181, 182, 195,
    215
Butt, D.S., 190, 215

Cairns, R.B., 149, 153, 215
Callaghan, J.W., 122, 184, 225
Callan, H., 128, 129, 215
Campbell, D.T., 175, 179, 195, 215,
    225
Candland, D.K., 28, 182, 189, 215
Cantor, N., 195, 215
Chalmers, N.R., 28, 31, 119, 215
Chance, M.R.A., 28, 41, 201, 215
Chapman, M., 157, 158, 221
Chapple, E.D., 41, 215

Chase, I.D., 175, 215
Cheska, A., 144, 215
Chrisjohn, R.D., 181, 222
Coe, C.L., 25, 222
Cofer, C.V., 144, 218
Coleman, J.S., viii, 123, 215
Coles, R., 9, 215
Collins, B.E., 23, 131, 215
Conger, J., 210, 215
Coombs, C., 11, 215
Coopersmith, S., 136, 215
Costa, P.T., 187, 215
Craik, K.H., 173, 177, 181, 182, 195, 215
Cronbach, L.J., 181, 216
Cronin, C.L., 125, 175, 206, 216, 225
Csikszentmihalyi, M., viii, x, 4, 140, 216
Cureton, E.E., 192, 217

Daly, M., 124, 125, 226
Darley, J., 170, 219
Darwin, C., 22, 24, 153, 216
Datta, S., 27, 29, 30, 218
David, D.S., 208, 216
Dawkins, R., 157, 216
Dehority, J., 196, 214
Demo, D.H., 3, 223
Dlugokinski, E.L., 174, 216
Dolhinow, P., 25, 216
Douvan, E., 123, 126, 216
Dovidio, J.F., 199, 216
Dumont, L., 29, 30, 216

Edelman, M.S., 175, 221
Edwards, C.P., 22, 170, 225
Eibl-Eibesfeldt, I., 14, 24, 202, 216
Eisenberg-Berg, N., 157, 170, 174, 182, 216, 220
Elder, G. Jr., 3, 5, 216
Elkins, H., 144, 216
Elliott, C., 40, 218
Ellyson, S.L., 199, 216
Endler, N.S., 173, 194, 216, 220
Epstein, S., 173, 181, 195, 216
Erikson, E.H., 14, 129, 193, 206, 216
Esser, A.H., 22, 23, 171, 211, 216
Eysenck, H.J., 181, 222

Farrell, W., 208, 216
Fekken, G.C., 181, 222
Felshin, J., 144, 216
Fine, G.A., 210, 211, 212, 216
Firestone, I.J., 174, 216
Fiske, D.W., 111, 175, 179, 190, 215, 218
Flannelly, K.J., 28, 217
Freedman, D.G., ix, 14, 23, 39, 41, 126, 153, 190, 199, 217, 221, 223
Freeman, M., 49, 221
Frenkel-Brunswik, E., 22, 213
Friedenberg, E., viii
Friedrich, L.K., 174, 217
Fulker, D.W., 181, 222

Gage, F.H., 28, 217
Gallagher, J.R., 47, 217
Garman, L., 196, 214
Gartlan, J.S., 27, 28, 217
Gauthreaux, S.A., Jr., 32, 33, 217
Gellert, E., 39, 141, 145, 217
Gibb, C.A., 22, 217
Gifford, R., 181, 217
Gilligan, C., 122, 129, 206, 210, 217
Glassner, B., 210, 211, 212, 216
Glidewell, J.C., 20, 21, 22, 213
Gold, M., 13, 23, 219
Golding, W., 17, 18, 217
Goodall, J., 198, 199, 217
Gordon, M.H., 192, 217
Gottman, J.M., 194, 217
Grinder, R.E., 1, 2, 5, 7, 9, 217
Groff, T.R., 13, 205, 225
Guthrie, R., 153, 217

Hall, E.T., 33, 217
Hall, G.S., vii, 9, 217
Hamburg, D.A, 201, 225
Hamilton, S.F., 2, 217
Hanson, E., 196, 214
Harrlow, R.N., 22, 219
Hartshorne, H., 174, 217
Hartup, W.W., 10, 122, 128, 157, 206, 217, 218
Harvey, O.J., 13, 20, 23, 49, 223
Hicks, B., 145, 218
Hill, J.P., 1, 2, 3, 4, 5, 6, 12, 173, 218

Hinde, R.A., 26, 27, 29, 30, 218
Hochschevender, M., 196, 214
Hoer, J.B., 28, 182, 189, 215
Hoffman, M., 127, 218
Holden, C., 13, 218
Hollingshead, A.B., vii, 12, 13, 47, 122, 123, 212, 218
Holloway, R.L., 210, 219
Holstein, C., 122, 218
Hood, W.R., 13, 20, 23, 49, 223
Horowitz, L., 49, 221
Hrdy, S.B., 210, 218
Hutt, C., 126, 218

Irwin, N., 49, 221
Itani, J., 32, 201, 218
Ivers, J.W., 123, 151, 225

Jaccard, J.J., 181, 218
Jacklin, C.N., 22, 124, 158, 170, 219
Jaquish, G.A., 11, 223
Jay, S.M., 40, 218
Jennings, J.R., 13, 219
Johnson, W.R., 144, 218
Jones, E.E., 11, 218
Jones, H.E., 11, 12, 218
Jones, L.V., 111, 218
Jones, M.C., 184, 220
Jorgensen, S.R., 3, 4, 5, 12, 218

Kamin, L.J., 207, 219
Kandel, D., 128, 218
Kantor, M.B., 20, 21, 22, 217
Kaplan, A., 124, 218
Kaplan, J.R., 31, 32, 218
Karlins, M., 22, 219
Katchadourian, H., 158, 218
Katz, P., 128, 158, 218
Keating, C., 184, 220
Kelley, H.H., 206, 219
Keller, M., 122, 223
Kelly, M., 122, 223
Kenyon, G., 144, 219
Kett, J., viii
Kiell, N., vii, 219
King, R., 159, 226
Kivlin, J.E., 144, 224

Klissouras, V., 184, 219
Koslin, B.L., 22, 218
Kreuz, L.E., 13, 219

Labouvie-Vief, G., 128, 225
Lacoste-Utamsing, C., de, 210, 219
Lamiell, J.T., 181, 219
Lancaster, J.B., 185, 219
Larson, R., viii, x, 4, 140, 216
Latane, B., 170, 219
Lebold, C., 196, 214
Leeds, A., 186, 219
Lenney, E., 147, 214
Lennon, R., 170, 216
Lerner, R.M., 1, 2, 3, 5, 6, 7, 219
Lesser, G., 128, 218
Levi-Strauss, C., 201, 219
Levinson, D., 22, 213
Lewontin, R.C., 207, 219
Linkey, H.E., 200, 225
Lippitt, R., 13, 21, 22, 23, 219
Livson, N., 3, 4, 5, 6, 10, 12, 174, 219
Loizos, C., 183, 219
Lorenz, K.Z., 24, 34, 219
Lott, D.F., 32, 219
Loveland, E.H., 192, 217
Loy, J.W., 144, 219

Maccoby, E.E., 22, 124, 158, 170, 219
MacDonald, K.B., 14, 15, 220
Magnusson, D., 173, 194, 216, 220
Maller, J.B., 174, 217
Marler, P., 35
Martyna, W., 147, 214
Marwell, G., 11, 225
Masters, R.D., 14, 220
Matza, D., 144, 220
Maxim, P.E., 28, 31, 32, 220
May, M.A., 174, 217
Mazur, A., 184, 220
Mazur, J., 184, 220
McCall, R., 196, 220
McCrae, R.R., 187, 215
McGrew, W.C., 46, 201, 220
McGuinness, D., 25, 28, 129, 201, 202, 207, 209, 220
McGuire, M.T., 33, 206, 220
McPherson, D., 144, 219

Mead, G.H., 144, 220
Mead, M., vii, 12, 122, 123, 220
Medin, D.L., 25, 220
Meek, L.H., 122, 123, 220
Mendoza, D.L., 124, 221
Mischel, M., 195, 215
Mischel, W., 173, 193, 195, 220
Mitchell, G., 25, 220
Morris, N.M., 13, 205, 225
Muczenski, D.M., 175, 184, 206, 225
Mussen, P., 157, 174, 182, 184, 220

Neale, M.C., 181, 222
Nisbet, R.E., 11, 218

Offer, D., viii
Olweus, D., 175, 220
Omark, D.R., x, 14, 45, 175, 184, 190,
    206, 220, 221, 225
Orne, M.T., 196, 221

Paikoff, R.L., ix, 132, 135, 221
Papania, D., 49, 221
Pargament, R., 22, 219
Parsons, T., 150, 221
Pattee, H.H., 29, 30, 221
Peskin, H., 3, 4, 5, 6, 10, 12, 174, 205,
    219, 221
Petersen, A.C., 4, 5, 221
Pitcairn, T.K., 198, 221
Pleck, J.H., 208, 209, 221
Plomin, R., 173, 215
Poirier, F.E., 32, 221
Polansky, N.W., 13, 21, 22, 23, 49,
    219, 221
Polsky, H.W., 211, 221
Postman, N., 9, 221
Pressley, M., 181, 222

Radke-Yarrow, M., 157, 158, 159, 221,
    226
Raj, M.H., 13, 205, 225
Ramirez, J.M., 124, 221
Rapaport, D., 49, 221
Raven, B.E., 23, 131, 215
Redican, W.K., 25, 221

Reitz, W., 136, 224
Richards, S.M., 27, 221
Riesen, A.H., 14, 221
Ringland, J.T., 194, 217
Roberts, J.M., 144, 221
Robinson, J., 136, 222
Rodgers, H.L., 122, 223
Rohr, R., 196, 214
Romer, N., 144, 222
Rose, R.M., 13, 219
Rose, S., 207, 219
Rosen, S., 13, 21, 22, 23, 219
Rosenblum, L.A., 25, 222, 224
Rowell, T.E., 28, 32, 34, 41, 222
Rushton, J.P., 157, 159, 174, 181, 222,
    224

Sade, D.S., 25, 29, 31, 34, 153, 222
Sarup, G., 122, 223
Sassen, G., 129, 222
Savin-Williams, R.C., ix, 3, 11, 25, 39,
    41, 42, 122, 126, 132, 135, 139,
    144, 145, 153, 157, 158, 164, 175,
    190, 199, 221, 222, 223, 226
Scheinfeld, D.R., 204, 223
Schneirla, T.C., 28, 223
Schoggen, P.S., 5, 26, 27, 223
Schwartz, R., 195, 223, 225
Schwartz, S., 136, 137, 139, 191, 192
Scott, J.P., 28, 223
Sechrest, L., 195, 225
Seyfarth, R.M., 28, 29, 119, 131, 223
Shaver, P., 136, 222
Shaw, viii
Sherif, C.W., 13, 20, 22, 23, 49, 122,
    184, 198, 202, 212, 223
Sherif, M., 13, 20, 23, 49, 184, 198,
    202, 212, 223
Shweder, R.A., 192, 223
Siegel, S., 48, 139, 223
Small, M.F., 34, 122, 185, 223
Small, S.A., ix, 157, 158, 164, 175,
    190, 223, 226
Smith, L.M., 20, 21, 22, 217
Smuts, B., 28, 119, 131, 223
Snyder, E.E., 144, 224
Sommer, R., 10, 194, 195, 196, 212,
    224
Southwick, C.M., 198, 224

Spinola, S.M., ix, 144, 223
Spreitzer, E., 144, 224
Stanford, R.N., 22, 213
Staub, E., 157, 174, 182, 224
Stein, A.H., 174, 217
Steinberg, L.D., 9, 224
Strayer, F.F., 14, 40, 42, 46, 90, 159, 197, 198, 221, 224
Stringer, L.A., 20, 21, 22, 217
Sullivan, J., 196, 214
Suttles, C.D., 13, 18, 224
Sutton-Smith, B., 144, 221
Swartz, K.B., 25, 224
Syme, G.J., 27, 224
Symons, D., 128, 224

Tanner, J.M., 47, 152, 158, 159, 224
Taub, D.M., 25, 221
Taylor, J., 136, 224
Thompson, C., 208, 224
Thompson, P.R., 14, 224
Thornburg, E.E., 2, 224
Thornburg, H.D., 2, 4, 5, 7, 12, 224
Thrasher, F., viii, 13, 18, 19, 202, 203, 204, 224
Tiger, L., 34, 128, 129, 224
Tinbergen, N., 9, 14, 22, 24, 34, 198, 212, 224, 225
Tittler, B., 122, 223
Tobin-Richards, M., 4, 5, 221
Torrance, E.P., 48, 225
Trivers, R.L., 157, 225

Udry, J.R., 13, 205, 225
Urberg, K., 128, 225

Vaughn, B.E., 175, 225

Wareing, S., 159, 224
Washburn, S.L., 201, 225
Waters, E., 175, 225
Watson, C., 147, 214
Waxler, C.Z., 170, 225
Webb, E., 195, 225
Wechsler, D., 48, 225
Weisfeld, C.C., 40, 122, 149, 175, 183, 184, 198, 201, 206, 225
Weisfeld, G.E., x, 15, 40, 122, 123, 149, 151, 157, 175, 183, 184, 198, 200, 201, 206, 225
Wells, L.E., 11, 225
Whaley, F., 49, 221
White, B.J., 13, 20, 23, 49, 223
Whiting, B., 22, 170, 225
Whyte, L.L., 29, 226
Wickler, W., 153, 226
Williams, R.C., 17, 214
Wilson, A.F., 29, 226
Wilson, D., 29, 226
Wilson, E.O., 28, 32, 33, 187, 226
Wilson, M., 124, 125, 226
Wright, H.F., 9, 26, 141, 160, 211, 213, 226

Yarrow, M.R., 170, 226
Yoshiba, K., 201, 226

Zahn-Waxler, C., 157, 158, 159, 221, 226
Zarit, S., 184, 226
Zeldin, R.S., ix, 157, 158, 164, 175, 190, 223, 226
Zuckerman, S., 34, 226

Subject Index

Activities, dominance interactions in, 108, 176

Adjective characterization, in camp adolescent study, 46–47

Adolescence, pubescence and, 204–207

Adolescence research
adolescence of, 1–3
conceptual issues in, 13–16
contextual quality of, 4
ethological perspective on, 14–16
intra-individual influences and, 5–6
life span and, 6
longitudinal, 3
methodological issues in, 8–13
multi-method/multi-trait/multi-variate analyses in, 3–4, 179–180
research agendas for, 1–8
theory-research-application balance in, 6–7
through eyes of adolescent, 4

Adolescent(s)
adolescence study through eyes of, 4
altruism in, 157–171

Advice
as act of dominance, 42, 171, 182
from female leaders, 115
from "maternal leaders," 114–115

Age
dominance ranking and, 86, 104, 112
as factor in dominance and social behavior, 131–156, 183

Aggression, 202
dominance hierarchy and suppression of, 209
as index of dominance, 175
in males, 206–207, 209

Alpha(s), 20, 37, 183, 186, 189, 198
assertive techniques of, 185, 203
characteristics of, 199–200
in lower class black groups, 204

Altruism and altruistic behavior
in adolescents, 157–171
definition of, 159–160
implications of, 168–171
individual consistency in, 161, 163
late adolescent females, 151
males, 158–164
mixed group, 164–171
nature of, 161
observation of, 175–180
peer rankings of, 160–161, 163, 165, 168, 171, 176, 177
self-report measure of, 190–191
sex differences in, 158, 166–168, 170
as a trait, 173–187

Amorphous Miss Average, characteristics of, 115

Antagonists, 198
in female groups, characteristics of, 115

Assistance behavior, in female sports group study, 146

Athletic ability
assessment of, 48
dominance ranking and, 59, 66, 77, 91, 104, 111, 112, 134
status in gangs and, 19

Athletic assessment, in camp adolescent study, 47

Athletic games
age and behavior in, 139–149, 153–156
dominance behavior in, 183

Attractiveness
    assessment of, 48
    dominance ranking and, 77, 111, 112
Avoidance behavior, in female sports
        group study, 146

Bed position
    determination of, 47
    dominance ranking and, 59, 66, 77,
        112, 133
    of female camp adolescents, 104
    of male camp adolescents, 59, 77
Bedtimes, dominance behavior, 108
Bem Sex Role Inventory, 146–147
Beneficiary categories, of helping behav-
        ior, 160
Benefits, of dominance heirarchy, 200–
    204
Beta, 37, 201
Biosocial perspective, of human behav-
        ior, 187
Body surface assessment, derivation of,
    47
Brains, in groups, characteristics of, 19
Bully(ies)
    dominance behavior of, 113–114, 183,
        198, 211
    in gangs, 19

California Psychological Inventory, 190
Camp experience, dominance behavior
        and, 134
Camp Wancaooah
    group dominance studies at, 37–50
    group geist at, 123–125
    setting of, 37–38
Camping ability
    peer ranking of, 177
    prosocial hierarchies and, 161
Camps, group hierarchal studies in, 20–
    22
Characteristics of individuals, dominance
        behavior and, 111–112
Cleanup periods, dominance behavior
        during, 108
Cohesive dyarchy
    effects of, 200–204
    in female group structure, 129, 150,
        210

Compliant Clingers, characteristics of,
    115–116, 200
Coopersmith Self-Esteem Inventory
    (SEI), 136
Counselor
    as receiver of helping behavior, 160
        in adolescent group, 162, 164,
        167
Counselor's favorites
    determination of, 48
    dominance behavior and, 112
Counselors-in-training, dominance behav-
        iors in, 132–135
Counter dominance behavior
    in camp adolescents, 58, 106, 110, 133
    indices of, 43
    in late adolescent females, 137
Crafts skills, dominance behavior and,
    134
Creativity
    assessment of, 48
    dominance behavior and, 112, 134
Cross-form stability, of dominance and
        altruism rankings, 177
Cross-situational stability, of prosocial
        and dominance behavior, 179

Delta, 37
Discussions, dominance behavior during,
    108, 133, 176, 183
Displacements, in dominance hierarchies,
    109–110
Distracting behavior, in female sports
        group study, 146
Dominance
    age as factor in, 131–156, 183
    athletic ability and, 184–185
    definition and measurement of, 27–28,
        39, 41
    self-report measure of, 190
    tests, measurements, and observations
        of, 47
    as a trait, 31, 173–187
Dominance behavior(s), 23
    analysis of observational data on, 43–
        44
    in camp groups, 20–22, 37–50
    characteristics of individual and, 111–
        112
    dyadic relationships and, 108–109

ethological perspective of, 17–35
extended studies of, 118–121
in female camp adolescents
    discussion of, 105–129, 203
    qualitative account of, 81–104
frequency of expression of, 106–108
in gangs, 18–21, 203, 204
group geist and, 123–125
group structure and, 109–111, 125,
    126
indices of, 42–43, 182
in late adolescent female group, 135–
    139
in male camp adolescents, 113–114
    discussion of, 105–129
    qualitative account of, 57–79
mode of expression of, 105–106
negative implications of, 23
prosocial hierarchies and, 161, 168
sex differences in, 170
sociological and social psychological
    studies of, 17–23
sociometric placings of, 45–47
styles of, 113–116
Dominance hierarchy, 30
    effects of, 200–204
    evolution of, 32–34
Dominance interactions, ethological stud-
    ies of, 27–35
Dominance rankings
    in female camp adolescent study, 85,
        91, 96–97, 103–104, 111
    in male camp adolescent study, 46, 59,
        65–66, 71, 77, 111
Dominance relationships, 29
    stability of, in late adolescent females,
        138
Dyadic relationships
    dominance behavior of, 62–63, 108–
        109, 185, 198
    in females, 129, 150

Ecological validity, of naturalistic re-
    search methods, 196–197
Encouragement behavior, in female sports
    group study, 146
Epsilon, 37
Ethological methodologies, psychological
    methodologies compared to, 190–
    192

Ethological studies, of adolescence, 14–
    16
Ethology
    definition of, 24
    of dominance interactions, 27–35
    human, 23–27
    methodological aspects of, 26–27
    nonhuman primate research and, 24–26
Evolution, of dominance hierarchies, 32–
    34
Expression of dominance
    frequency of, 106–108
    mode of, 105–106
Extended studies, of dominance, 118–121

Female cabin groups
    life in, 81–104
    mode of dominance behavior in, 103–
        106, 114–118
Female contingency hypothesis, 128
Female adolescent groups
    altruistic behavior in, 151, 164–171
    behavioral interactions in, 121–123
    dominance behavior in, 103–106, 114–
        118, 209–210
    athletic ability related to, 184–185
Female volleyball games, dominance be-
    havior studies on, 144–149
Fights, in cabin groups, 54, 105, 203
Free time
    dominance behavior during, 176
    prosocial behavior during, 162, 164
Friendship rankings
    in camp adolescent study, 46, 59
    prosocial hierarchies and, 161
Friendship traits, in camp adolescent
    study, 46
Funny Boy
    in groups, 204
    characteristics of, 19

Gamma, 37
Gangs
    dominance behavior in, 18–21, 203–
        204
    roles in, 204
Genetics
    male aggression and, 206–207
    male sex role stereotypes and, 208

Gentle men, 207–210
Goat
    in groups, 204
    characteristics of, 19
Gossip, as dominance behavior, 42, 90
Group, as receiver of helping behavior,
        160, 162, 164, 167
Group activities, prosocial behavior of
        adolescents in, 162, 164
Group-dominance study on camp adoles-
        cents, 37–50
    female cabin groups, 81–104
    human subjects in, 49–50
    male cabin groups, 51–79
    observational data from, 41–44, 58–59
    participant description, 38–39
    pilot study for, 39–41
    procedures used in, 41–49
    setting of, 37–38
    sociometric placings in, 45–47
    tests and measurements used in, 47–48
Group geist, among camp adolescents,
        123–125
Group hierarchy, in summer camps, 20–
        21
Group roles, 19
Group structure
    dominance behavior and, 109–111,
        125–126
    methodological perspectives of, 197–
        199
    observations on in male camp, 132
    sociometrics of, 133

Harvard Step Test, 48
Helpers, high and low, in adolescent pro-
        social behavior study, 163–164,
        169–170
Hierarchy, concept of, 29–30
Hiking position
    assessment of, 48
    dominance ranking and, 59, 77, 112, 134
Hollingshead's index of socioeconomic
        status, 47
Homosexuality, 52, 54, 55, 60, 94, 98,
        100, 109, 144
Hormones, adolescent sexual behavior
        and, 13, 205
Humans, dominance and submissive be-
        haviors in, 34

"Idiosyncratic male hypothesis," 206
Individual activities, prosocial behavior
        of adolescents in, 162, 164
Individual and family characteristics,
        methods for obtaining, 47–48
Intelligence
    determination of, 48
    dominance ranking and, 66, 86, 104,
        112, 134
Interaction frequency, dominance behav-
        ior and, 134
Intimacy, male perception as threat, 129
Involvement, dominance behavior and,
        112

Jokers, dominance behavior of, 114
Jokes
    in female cabin life, 98, 104
    in male cabin life, 51–52, 61

Late adolescent females, dominance be-
        havior study on, 135–139
Leader(s), in gangs, 19, 204
Leadership, observation of, 48
Leadership traits
    in camp adolescent study, 46, 127
    dominance ranking and, 97, 111, 112,
        134, 201
Life span, adolescence research and, 6
Longitudinal research, on adolescence, 3
Lord of the Flies, competitive adolescent
        behavior in, 17–18

Male bonding theory, 128
Male cabin groups
    life in, 51–79
    mode of dominance behavior in, 103–
        104, 113–114, 116–117
Male counselors-in-training, behavioral
        dominance hierarchy in, 133–135
Male gender, sex role stereotypes and,
        208–209
Male volleyball games, dominance be-
        havior studies on, 139–143
"Maternal Leader(s)," 92
    characteristics of, 114–115
Mealtimes, dominance behavior during,
        108, 133, 137, 176

Men's Movement, 189, 207–210
"Minnesota Twins" research project, 13
Multi-method/multi-trait/multi-variate
    analysis
    in adolescence research, 3–4
    of altruism and dominance behavior
        data, 179–180

Naturalistic observations, of personality
    phenomena, 194–196
Negative expression behavior, in female
    sports group study, 146
Nonhuman primate research, human
    ethology and, 24–26

Omega(s), 37, 109, 186, 189, 198, 211
    characteristics of, 201, 202
Outcamping ability, dominance behavior
    and, 134
Overtness
    assessment of, 47
    dominance behavior and, 70, 105–106,
        112, 134, 137, 138–139, 183

Participant observers, of human behavior,
    benefits and problems from, 210–
    212
Peer(s)
    camp group structure assessment by,
        22
    as receiver of helping behavior, 160
    in adolescent group, 162, 164, 167
Peer friendship, dominance behavior and,
    134, 151
Peer leaders, dominance behavior of, 113
Peer rankings
    of altruism, 160–161, 163, 165, 168,
        171, 176, 177
    temporal stability of, 179
Peer rating studies, in late adolescent fe-
    males, 139
Personality, dominance behavior and, 183
Physical assertion behavior
    in female camp adolescents, 103, 106,
        110, 151
    indices of, 42
    in male camp adolescents, 65, 106,
        110, 133

Physical assistance
    as form of altruism, 159
    in adolescent groups, 162, 164, 166,
        168
Physical or object displacement behavior
    in female camp adolescents, 90, 105,
        106, 110
    indices of, 43
    in made camp adolescents, 65, 71, 76,
        105, 106, 110, 133
Physical fitness
    assessment of, 48
    dominance ranking and, 59, 66, 112
Physical serving
    as form of altruism, 159
    in adolescent groups, 162, 164
Physical size, dominance ranking and,
    77, 86, 97, 112, 134
Popularity
    dominance behavior and, 112
    peer ranking of, 177
Problem campers, dominance encounters
    in, 92
Prosocial behavior, see Altruism and al-
    truistic behavior
Psychological methodologies, ethological
    methodologies compared to, 190–
    192
Pubertal development
    assessment of, 47
    dominance ranking and, 66, 77, 91,
        111, 112, 134, 151–152
Pubescence, adolescence and, 204–207

Quiet Followers, dominance behavior of,
    114

Rank order, see Dominance rankings
Recognition behavior
    in female camp adolescents, 85, 90,
        105, 106, 110, 137
    indices of, 42–43
    in male camp adolescents, 65, 71, 76,
        106, 110, 133
Reliability checks, on dominance behav-
    ior observations, 44–45
Research agendas
    review of, 1–7
    setting of, 7–8

Rest periods, dominance behavior in,
    108, 183
Reversal rates, of dominance behaviors,
    137

Schwartz Ascription of Responsibility
    Scale, 136, 191
Self esteem
    dominance behavior and, 136, 139,
        151
    prosocial hierarchies and, 161, 168,
        177
Self-reports, in assessing personality phe-
    nomena, 190, 193–194
Sex differences
    in adolescent prosocial activity, 166–
        168
    in dominance hierarchies, 126–129, 183
Sex-role hypothesis, age differences in
    sports behaviors and, 149
Sex- role stereotypes, of males, 208–209
Sexual behavior in adolescents, hormones
    and, 13, 205
Sharing
    as form of altruism, 159
    in adolescent groups, 162, 164, 166,
        168
Show-Off
    in groups, 204
    characteristics of, 19
Sissy
    in groups, 204
    characteristics of, 19–22
Sit beside behavior
    dominance behavior and, 112
    observation of, 48
Social behavior, age as factor in, 131–
    156
Social status, biological pubescence and,
    205–206
Socioeconomic status
    determination of, 47
    dominance ranking and, 77, 111, 112,
        134
Socioempathy
    assessment of, 47
    dominance behavior and, 112
Sociometric placings, of dominance be-
    havior, 45–47

Sociometric studies, of power dynamics
    in summer camp, 21, 45–47
Spirit, dominance behavior and, 134
Sports behavior, age trends in, 153–156
Stabilization, of group structure, 203
Status, in gangs, 19
Submission, styles of, 114, 115–116
Submissive Followers, characteristics of,
    114, 200
Subordination
    benefits of, 33, 202
    gestures in, 88
    reaction patterns in, 186
Subtle dominance behavior, 183

Tanner's Pubertal Maturational Scale,
    159
Temporal stability, of prosocial and dom-
    inance behaviors, 178–179
Theory-research-application balance, in
    adolescence research, 6–7
Torrance Test of Creativity, 48
Traits, dominance and altruism as, 173–
    187
Travel camp sessions, prosocial behavior
    studies on, 176–177
Twins, altruism studies on, 181

Verbal assistance
    as form of altruism, 159
    in adolescent groups, 162, 164, 166,
        168
Verbal control behavior
    in female camp adolescents, 103, 106,
        110, 137
    indices of, 43
    in male camp adolescents, 71, 106,
        110, 133
Verbal directive behavior
    in female camp adolescents, 85, 86,
        90, 91, 106, 110
    indices of, 42
    in male camp adolescents, 58, 59, 70,
        71, 106, 110, 133
Verbal or physical threat behavior, 183
    in female camp adolescents, 90, 105,
        106, 110
    indices of, 43

in male camp adolescents, 90, 105,
        106, 110
Verbal ridicule behavior
  in female camp adolescents, 85, 90,
        91, 96, 103, 105, 106, 110, 137
  indices of, 42
  in male camp adolescents, 58, 65, 70,
        71, 76, 103, 105, 106, 110, 133
Verbal support
  as form of altruism, 159
    in adolescent groups, 162, 164, 166

Volleyball games
  dominance behavior studies on, 201
    female players, 144–149
    male players, 139–143, 198

Wilderness trips, adolescent prosocial be-
        havior studies on, 157–171
WISC test, 48